Juggling -

WHAT IT IS AND HOW TO DO IT:

A NOT-SO-BRIEF INTRODUCTION TO THE
WORLD'S MOST UNDERRATED PASTIME

Thom Wall

Modern Vaudeville Press
PHILADELPHIA, PA

Modern Vaudeville Press
113 E. Mayland St.
Philadelphia, PA 19144
USA
www.modernvaudevillepress.com
info@modernvaudevillepress.com

Photographs by Avi Pryntz-Nadworny—www.photopryntz.com

Photos modeled by Benjamin Domask-Ruh—www.benjamindomask.com

Edited by Benjamin Domask-Ruh and Carly Schuna

Ordering Information:
Quantity sales. Special discounts are available on quantity purchases by corporations, associations, and others. For details, contact the "Special Sales Department" at the address above.

Juggling: What It Is and How to Do It / Thom Wall. —1st ed.
ISBN 978-1-7339712-5-6

Dedicated to Jim Hendricks

and the entire St. Louis neverthriving

for giving me the life I have today.

Juggling: The only hard parts are the throwing and the catching.

- John Teasdale, British juggler and mathematician

CONTENTS

FOREWORD

YEARS BEFORE I MET THOM, I taught myself to juggle when I was about 12 years old, using baseballs I had laying around in my room. It took me about a day, and upon successfully doing about 10 throws of the cascade, I put the balls down...for 15 years.

I really learned how to juggle from a book. I bought *Charlie Dancey's Encyclopaedia of Ball Juggling* at a store across the street from the Japanese Consulate in Chicago, which was where I was working at the time. I bought the book, bought some More Balls Than Most balls, and took everything back to my apartment. I had never realized that the tricks had names, or that there were so many tricks to learn. I resolved to check off as many tricks as I could master. I started joining Tony Flowers and company down at the Oak Street Beach hangout on weekends. Six years later, I had a silver medal in the IJA Stage Championships and I was invited to train the Cirque du Soleil *Quidam* diabolo troupe. All this...from a book.

Now, 23 years later, I look back on that fateful purchase and I laugh out of joy at how my life has changed. People met. Feelings felt. Places seen. All because I bought a book. One place I got to go in 2008 was Washington University in St. Louis where a young college lad named Thom Wall was hosting a festival together with his juggling club. Watching Thom and his minions on Friday afternoon stick funny names for each full bore trophy for the games on Sunday gave me a warm feeling of anticipation. Indeed, the festival was a killer, and I remember writing in my review of the festival, "Thom Wall—this guy should run the IJA festival. No joke."

In the 12 years that have followed, I have seen Thom be elected to the IJA Board (a gig that is sometimes tougher than running the IJA Festival), win his own IJA silver medal, go on tour with Cirque du Soleil for five years as a main act, and publish two very excellent books on juggling (one of which you are now holding in your hand).

I am a Japanese teacher, so I use the terms *senpai/kouhai* in reference to someone who is a mentor and someone who is mentored. And while I started before Thom, and came up in the game before him, he is clearly my *senpai*. He is the pro and I am the pretender. He actually KNOWS what he's talking about, because he has lived it. When Thom asked me to read his book and write the foreword, I was honored, because this was THOM WALL asking little ol' me for help. And you know what? I learned some new things from this book. At a point in my juggling life where I pretty much thought I knew what I knew and there was little else to discover, Thom—as a *senpai* should—taught me the error of my ways. There are things in this book that I'm going to apply to my practice TOMORROW. I'm going to try to crack that pesky balance-with-a-juggle problem I've always had using this book. Old dogs and new tricks indeed.

So there it is. The book you're holding will help you become a better juggler—full stop. No matter where you are on your own path, this book and Thom's careful, conscientious and research-based instruction will take you further down that path. Most juggling books tell you how to learn a particular trick, whereas Thom has taken that approach further by teaching you how to learn ANY trick. And, icing on the cake, his approach is scholarly and based in science, rather than simply anchored in anecdote and personal experience. You know, the whole give a man a fish vs. teaching how to fish. Thom is not only telling you what bait to use and how long your pole should be; he's telling you WHY those instructions are efficacious and valid. Sign me up.

It bears repeating that when you buy a book, you can never be sure where it will take you and what impact it will have on your life. All I would suggest at this point is that you read and use this book well, because Thom-*senpai* is dropping some serious knowledge, and while I don't know much, I do know the goods when it comes to good instruction and deep juggling knowledge. Thom has the goods, and he wants to pass it on to you. In fact, you're holding it in your hands. What are you waiting for? Turn the page and get on it!

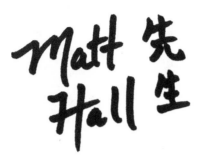

Matt Hall
Palo Alto, California, USA
March 2020

PREFACE

I STARTED WRITING this book in 2016, when I was on tour with Cirque du Soleil in Japan. While I was working for them there—as well as later on in Belgium, Spain, France and beyond—I taught a juggling class to the show's ushers and front-of-house staff. This enthusiastic group of new friends was my respite—a break from the grind of 10-show weeks and a breath of fresh air. This was a group of people who showed up every week, bright-eyed and excited about learning a new skill—people who genuinely cared about the art of juggling and the learning process. I owe them a debt of gratitude.

I would like to extend a very special thank-you to Benjamin Domask-Ruh. He went over this book with a fine-tooth comb in its final stages and offered support and encouragement throughout the entire writing process. This book would not have happened without this wonderful clown, colleague, and friend.

This book is structured the same way that I teach my private students. We move from learning the fundamentals to understanding the theory behind juggling. Along the way, other techniques, such as balance and inventing new tricks, are introduced. Finally, we talk about act creation and how to apply your new skills in ways that an audience would enjoy.

Feel free to move through this book from chapter to chapter—or to jump around and work on what seems most enjoyable to you. Enthusiasm is the key to learning anything, and I hope this book will motivate you to train hard and teach you how to train smart.

Juggling, as a performance art and as a hobby, has been a source of inspiration and comfort for me throughout my life. I sincerely hope it has a similarly profound impact on you.

Good luck! Have fun!

Thom Wall
Philadelphia, Pennsylvania, USA
March 2020

A FEW NOTES ON DIAGRAMS

IN THE FOLLOWING CHAPTERS, a variety of different diagrams and styles will be used. Each pattern will be explained in three different ways—a step-by-step cartoon, a ladder diagram, and a long-exposure photograph taken with LED balls. This has been done in an attempt to make this book useful to aspiring jugglers with different learning modalities.

The cartoons offer snapshots of what the pattern looks like at different points in time. These points in time are called "beats."

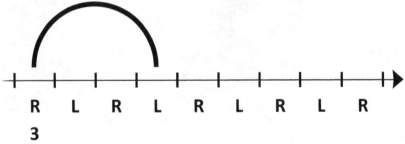

4   4   1

This diagram explains the pattern 441. You'll see this diagram— as well as many others—in later chapters.

Ladder diagrams show the mathematical relationship between each throw and catch over time—when objects are thrown and when they return to hands.

R   L   R   L   R   L   R   L   R

3

This ladder diagram shows how a three-beat throw goes from one hand to the other. The vertical dashes represent divisions in time.

Note that the dashes represent the division of time into "beats." This is the most mathematically intense diagrammatic style in this book. If it is not immediately understandable, don't panic! Ladder diagrams are not always immediately understandable to all learning styles. Appendix 1 explains siteswap notation, which will give you a robust understanding of this kind of diagram.

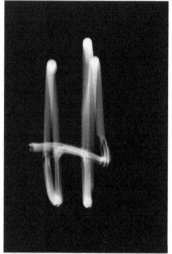

The long-exposure images allow a learner to see the full "topography" of the pattern in a single image.

This photograph shows the shape of the juggling pattern 441.

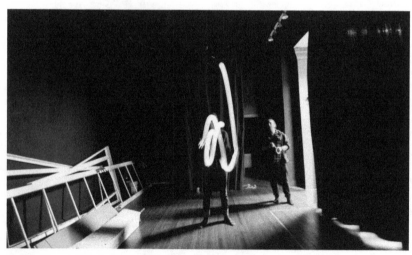

Behind the scenes with Benjamin Domask-Ruh and Avi Pryntz-Nadworny. Here, Thom is about to place spike tape, marking Benjamin's feet before taking photographs for this book.

ELEMENTS OF SUCCESSFUL JUGGLING

WHEN YOU START, juggling three objects will seem like an impossible task. There are more objects than you have hands, and you need to control them all at once! What's the secret? How is it possible? It's all so overwhelming!

Juggling as a whole is unlike other circus disciplines. Learning to tumble or dance on the trapeze can rely on brute strength and lighting-fast reflexes. Juggling, on the other hand, is almost entirely a mental game. In many ways, learning to juggle is more about cultivating the relationship between your body and objects and the relationship between your body and time than it is about physical strength or daring.

The first pattern you learn when you juggle three balls is called the *three-ball cascade*. It's a symmetrical pattern where all of the objects cross at a point in the middle and all of the throws you make are the same. By breaking the pattern down from "three objects and two hands, and there's so much going on, and there's no time!" to the much more digestible "training a single throw," you're able to focus on other aspects of our intial juggling pattern. At its core, juggling is about learning to focus on just one thing at a time. Every pattern can be broken down into single elements, which can be trained independently of one another.

In order to achieve a "successful" juggling pattern, you must master a few different variables. These elements include:

Consistency in height: All throws reach the same maximum height in their trajectory.

Consistency in width: The pattern is approximately as wide as the shoulders.

Consistency in crossing point: Since the throws all have the same height and width, their trajectories always intersect in the same point in space.[1]

Consistency in rhythm: Balls are thrown and caught on an even tempo, always alternating left and right.

Throws and catches are made low: Balls are thrown and caught low, near the navel.

The hands move in a circle: This circular motion of the hands, known as the "scoop," is what permits the balls to travel in the horizontal plane.

THE WINDOW

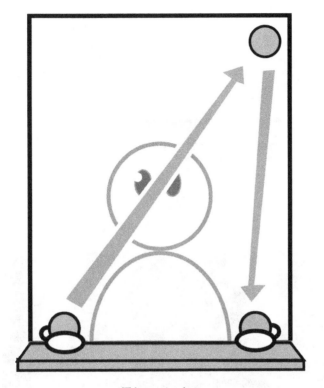

The window

IMAGINE YOU ARE STANDING in front of a window, with your hands resting on the sill at navel height. The sides of the window raise up—as wide as your shoulders—eventually making a corner with the window's top edge, some two feet above your sight line.

When we throw the ball in a three-object cascade, we're throwing from one hand, up and across to the opposite corner. The ball then descends down the side of the window—our shoulder line—and lands in the opposite hand. The hand never raises above the bottom of the sternum.

Our hand makes a "scooping" motion, making catches outside of the shoulder line and releasing the throw on the inside of the shoulder line.

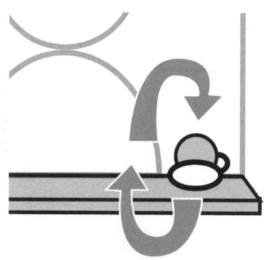

*The outward-to-inward rotation of
the scoop motion*

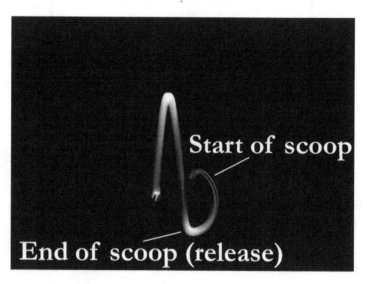

The scoop is the most fundamentally important part of juggling. When you watch seasoned pros juggling seven or eight or even 13 objects, you'll notice their hands always follow this scooping pattern. The scoop is what allows the ball to travel in a horizontal plane, rather than moving forwards (forcing you to walk forwards and chase the ball), or backwards (over your head)!

Your feet should be shoulder-width apart, giving you a nice solid base to work with.[2]

This scoop is your major C. It's the line in your handstand, the salt on your french fries, the cream in your coffee.[3] It's the basis of everything that we'll be doing and the thing that makes juggling work effectively. Of course, we'll break some of these rules later on—for now, just understand that it's a very important thing to be aware of.

The scoop is often represented (and, indeed, explained!) as a circle. This is a great way to think about it, but be aware that as you become more efficient with your motions, it will likely change to be more triangular in shape. Don't fret! In many places in this book, a triangle will be used to demonstrate this scooping motion. The most important thing to be aware of is the outward-to-inward movement of the hand along this pathway.

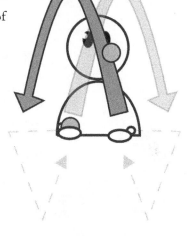

---

2 This shoulder-width stance has been a "best practice" in the juggling world for ages but was recently given scientific credence. In 2016, a research group from São Paulo State University published a paper called "Postural Control During Cascade Ball Juggling: Effects of Expertise and Base of Support", where they found that intermediate jugglers with their legs closer than shoulder width were more prone to body sway and errors in their juggling pattern than a similarly skilled group with a shoulder-width stance (Rodrigues, Polastri, Gotardi, & Barbieri, 2016).

These researchers found a correlation between postural control and expert juggling—let's put their theory to practice!

3 I take mine black, though, if you're buying!

GETTING STARTED WITH THREE BALLS

The First Throw

THE REAL SECRET to juggling three is that all of the throws are exactly the same. As we saw earlier, they all have the same height, they're all thrown at the same rhythm, and they all cross in the same point in space. When you're doing one-ball drills, you're really juggling three balls... just with two fewer balls.

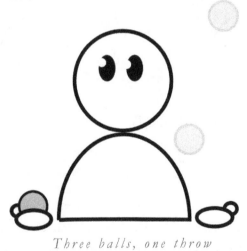

Three balls, one throw

Drill: Three-Ball Juggling with Just One Ball

This drill is a perfect way to start learning good form—that is, good throw placement and hand scoop—burning the pattern into your body's memory and setting yourself up for success when we add more balls.

Stand in place, with your feet shoulder-width apart. Your arms are bent at the elbows, slightly apart from your body—imagine you're holding a large box. Imagine the "corners" of the window above the shoulder-line.

Throw the ball from one hand to the other, making sure it passes through the corner of our window. Our throwing hand makes a proper scooping motion. Our catching hand does not reach up to make the catch.

This drill isn't a race—we are focusing on proper throw height, placement, and the scooping motion here. We'll get to tempo soon enough. Don't worry about making the next throw immediately upon catching the first ball. Take a breath, get settled, and make the next throw.

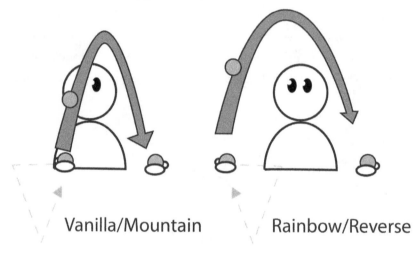

Vanilla/Mountain   Rainbow/Reverse

Mountains vs. Rainbows

Note: Mountains, not rainbows! Are you making a proper hand scoop? If you are, the throws will look like a mountain. They should be low in the center and peak in the corner. If the throws look like rainbows—low on the sides and tall in the middle—you're probably releasing the ball too early. Make sure you're releasing the throw at the end of the scoop![4]

---

4 There's no rule in juggling that says this is the "only" way to learn. In fact, there are hardly any rules in juggling at all (some would argue that there isn't a single one!) It's entirely possible to learn with just about any technique. This book focuses on "standard"

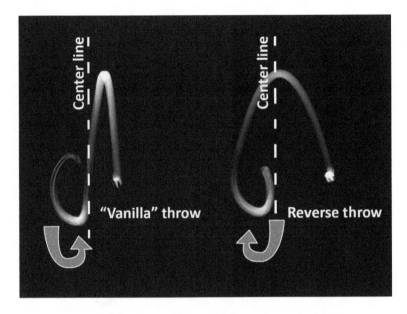

Drill: Throw, Throw, Catch, Catch

(...or, when we start, "throw, throw, drop, drop")

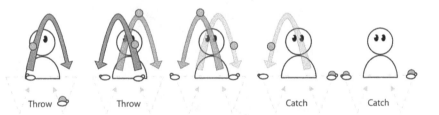

Throw   Throw   Catch   Catch

The first step of this drill is learning the appropriate timing for the second throw. The second throw should leave the hand when the first throw is reaching zero velocity—that moment in the ball's trajectory where it hangs in the air, about to fall back toward Earth.

Remember, these throws are made on their own independent beats. It might be helpful to say the words out loud—"throw, throw, catch, catch"—to get a better feel for your timing.

---

juggling technique in North America, which revolves around scoops and siteswaps. We're setting rules now so we can break them more easily as this book moves forward.

The brain likes to make things efficient by lumping motions together. If the balls are falling at more or less the same time, it's possible that you're making the throws at the same time. If you find yourself doing this, you need to iron out the mistake immediately. Training this way will set you back quite a bit and hinder your development when you try to add the third ball.

Practice this drill starting with both hands. Once you can get 10 successful attempts back-to-back, you're ready to add the third ball. If you find the second ball doesn't go high enough (so the first throw is a nice, tall throw and the second one is low and rushed), think about making the second throw taller than the first one—past the first ball's apex.

Where to Look

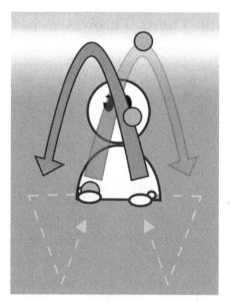

Focus on the top of the pattern

Hold up! Before we add that third throw, let's talk about focus. When we add the second throw, new jugglers often wonder where to look. Tracking multiple objects at the same time is tricky business!

The short answer: Look at a spot in the middle of the pattern, toward the top.

The long answer: As we mentioned earlier, the practice of juggling enhances the body's ability to interpret information in the periphery of the visual field—to understand the movement of objects without focusing on them directly (Draganski, Gaser, Busch, Schuierer, & Bogdahn, 2004). Though you may be tempted to try and focus on each ball, one at a time, the most effective place to look when juggling is the top of the pattern, in the center (Amazeen, Amazeen, Post, & Beek, 1999). This allows you to attend to all of the balls at the same time, rather than shifting your attention from one object to another (Cavanagh & Alvarez, 2005).

The idea of a "fixed gaze" in juggling was studied in 2011 by a team of researchers from the Netherlands. They found that expert jugglers executed patterns with greater throw consistency when they fixed their gaze towards the top of the juggling pattern rather than shifting focus. The study also noted that novice jugglers would have variability in their throws regardless of focus—but indicated that as jugglers' technique improved, their gaze began to shift from individual balls to the pattern as a whole (Dessing, Frederic, & Beek, 2011). Gazing "through" the pattern in this way provides the juggler with a constant visual reference point—a fixed background in juggler's vision acts as a landmark and allows for greater consistency of throws (Leigh & Zee, 2006) (Morisita & Yagi, 2001) (Byrne & Crawford, 2010).

In other words: *For juggling success, look at the whole pattern instead of individual objects.*[5]

The top of the balls' trajectories contain the most useful information for the juggler. With very little practice, your body will understand where the balls are going to land and make the catches for you. In a 2013 study

---

5 This said, know that it will take some time to be able to shift your focus from each individual ball to the pattern as a whole! Like everything else in juggling, this is a game of practice.

at the Research Institute for Sport and Exercise Sciences at Liverpool John Moores University in England, researchers determined that jugglers don't need to have the lower half of their visual field at all to proficiently juggle three balls–they determined that the source of information is the top half of the juggling pattern, and that success in three-ball juggling for beginners can also be measured by the heights of their throws (Sanchez Garcia, Hayes, Williams, & Bennett, 2013).

If you're worried about not focusing on each ball, don't be! So long as they're in your visual field, you'll be fine. In fact, you don't even need the bottom half of your visual field to juggle—you only need to see two percent of a ball for your brain to calculate exactly where it will end up. This is true for both expert and novice jugglers (Sanchez Garcia, Hayes, Williams, & Bennett, 2013).

Drill: The Third Throw

You've made 10 successful back-to-back attempts at the two-ball drill? Great! It's time to add that third ball.

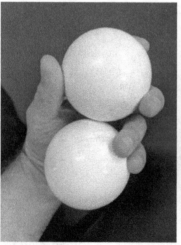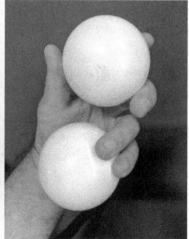

Hold two balls in one hand like this—the balls are gripped with different parts of the hand and can be manipulated independently. These photos are of the same hand, gripping the same balls in the same way. Notice how the hand can control each ball independently by curling and extending the fingers and palm.

To begin with, we'll hold two balls in your dominant hand and one ball in the non-dominant hand. When we hold two balls in one hand, there's one held in the palm and another in the fingers. The ball in the fingers is the first one that will be thrown in a three-ball pattern.

Three-ball juggling is the same as the two-ball drill that we just did, only with an extra ball. When the first throw is at its peak, we throw the second ball. When that one is at its peak, we make the third throw.

Remember: When we start with three balls, we need two in one hand and one in the other. We always start with the hand with two balls, and the first throw is the ball held by the thumb and forefingers.

Drill: "Throw, Throw, Get Rid of It!"

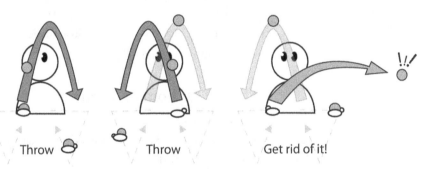

Throw   Throw   Get rid of it!

Learning to throw the third ball is often considered the hardest step when learning to juggle three balls—however, most new jugglers don't train the foundational drills outlined in this book. If you've been practicing everything outlined so far, you're in great shape!

"Throw, throw, get rid of it" is a way to teach your body to activate the third throwing motion and break the habit we've been building—making two throws and stopping.

Making a beautiful, well-spaced, accurate throw with that third ball might be a tall order for your first attempt. On your first try of this drill, just make a point of getting rid of that third ball at the appropriate time. It doesn't matter if it's caught or not—we're defining success as simply activating the throwing motion with the third ball at the appropriate time.

Slowly but surely, we'll "shape" that throw to be perfect.[6] The timing of this new toss should be as follows: throw, throw, catch, *throw!*

After you've done the "get rid of it" drill a few times successfully, it's time to change the exercise slightly. The adage in juggling is *perfect throws make perfect catches*—we're not worried about making the catch so much as we are about making a perfect throw.

Make the first two throws as you have been, but put your mental energy into that third ball—making sure that it's executed at the right time (as we did in the last drill), and placed appropriately in space. Don't worry about making the first two catches—just focus on the third ball's placement. If it's perfect, the catch will take care of itself. Work on this drill for a while, and once you're experiencing success with it, put some of your thought into catching the first two balls as well as the third. Once you've achieved three throws and catches—congratulations! You've just made your first three-ball flash.[7] You're officially a juggler!

Drill: The Fourth Throw

Remember when I said that the third throw was often considered the hardest part? I was lying. Sorry about that.

Our newest challenge is to make the fourth throw. You've been teaching your body and brain to stop after the third throw with every drill we've

---

6 This idea of "general to specific"—that is, the idea of getting the basic fundamental of "throwing at a particular time" and working toward "throwing at a particular time, to a particular place"—is a core concept in the fine arts. This approach allows you to start be seeing the wider idea—the "large, generalized form" as a foundation upon which more specific attention can be given (Rockman, 2000). We'll follow this approach through most of the book, referring to it as "shaping"—where we go from the broad idea first—either timing, direction, placement, or another variable, adding other elements as we move forward.

7 In juggling parlance, a "flash" is a string of throws and catches equal to the number of objects being juggled. In the context of three-ball juggling, three throws and three catches is called a "three-ball flash." A run of throws and catches that's double the number of objects being juggled—so, six throws and six catches of three-ball juggling—is called a "qualify."

done so far. It's time to break that pattern and make one more throw. (Don't panic! You've totally got this!)

To learn the fourth throw, we go back to the old "get rid of it!" drill… only now, it's "throw, throw, throw, get rid of it!" We're not worried about the shape or the placement of the fourth throw, just that your body activates the throwing motion at the right time.

Once you've experienced success with activating the fourth throw, shift some focus back to the placement. A perfect throw means a perfect catch—see if you can achieve a "run" of four catches of three-ball juggling without dropping![8]

Drill: The Fifth Throw (go for Six!)

For the fifth, sixth, seventh, and thousandth throws, the exercise is more or less the same. Force your body to make the new throw, then eventually shift your focus to the throw's placement. Remember, timing the throw is the most important aspect when learning to juggle. It doesn't matter how perfect your throws are if they're made at the wrong time.

After you make your sixth throw, the name of the game is practice. Through repetition, you'll start burning the motion of the throws into your body and mind. After your first six throws and catches, you'll soon get 10, then 15, 20, 30, 50, and eventually hundreds and hundreds of throws and catches in a single run.[9]

For now, though, it's time to put down this book and get to work! The rest of this book will make a lot more sense when you start putting what you've read so far into practice!

---

8 …but remember, drops simply mean that you're trying something new! Don't get discouraged—just pick up the balls and try again!

9 It's actually a scientific fact that the more you practice three-ball juggling as a beginner, the more quickly you'll achieve success. In a 2004 study, a group of researchers found that learners' increase in number of catches as they practiced over a four-week period was literally *exponential*. This was attributed to their changing form ("the appropriate kinematics")—that is, successful scooping motions – as their training progressed (Haibach, Daniels, & Newell, 2004).

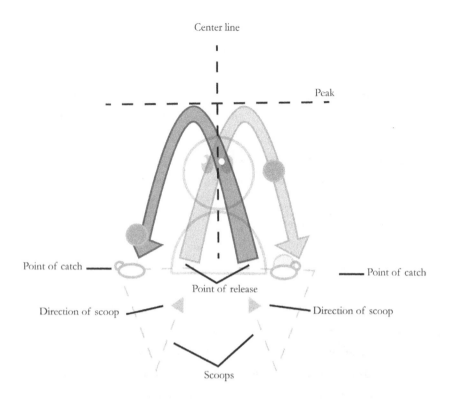

Time for a Quick Recap!

We've been over a lot of material so far. If you're having issues, remember that our three-ball cascade is built out of the following elements:

• Our hands move in circles, or "scoops," that move from the outside to the inside.

• Our hands catch on the outermost point of the scoop and throw/ release on the innermost point of the scoop.

• Objects cross at a point along the center line of the body.

• Objects all reach the same height, peaking in the top of our line of sight.

• Throws come from alternate hands: Right, left, right, left...

COMMON MISTAKES (AND HOW TO STOP DOING THEM.)

Problem: Walking Forward

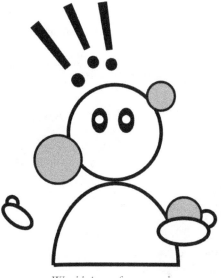

Walking forward

Walking forward, chasing the pattern as you juggle it, is a symptom of one or two things.

As we mentioned before, it can be the product of a faulty scoop. If you're catapulting the ball—that is, the ball is launched by the force of your elbow hinging—these errant throws can often happen. Catapults don't launch things from side to side; they launch objects in a perpendicular axis.

Chasing the balls can also be a product of narrow throws. If your throws aren't travelling all the way to the line of the opposite shoulder, the next throw is forced to sneak inside of it to make the next throw—tight to your chest. This distorts the shape of the scoop, resulting in a throw that is released in a forward motion. Make sure your scooping motion goes from side-to-side, parallel to your shoulders, rather than front-to-back.

If you're finding that your juggling pattern makes you walk, pay attention to the width of the throws and the movement of your hands. Practicing while facing a wall is a great drill to help iron out these kinks. Your brain might trick you into thinking you're juggling without walking, and a brick wall is an excellent tool to keep you honest.[10]

This can also be the result of a pattern that's too slow. If you're not making each throw when the one before it is reaching its apex, you can run into issues. Does it feel like each catch is being made as the throw before it is being caught, so you almost have two balls in a single hand as you make an exchange? If so, this might be your issue.

Problem: Hands Moving Up

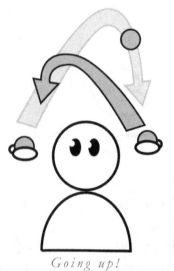

Going up!

If your hands are moving up while you juggle, it's probably the result of one of two things: Either you're too eager to make the next catch or you're just plain freaking out. (There's a lot going on here! I understand!)

Odds are, if your hands race upward when you start juggling, you're thinking way too much about catching. The timing of the throws might feel right to you—it's a relief to get them out of your hands

---

10 This said, don't rely on walls as your primary method of training! A 1998 study from the University of Wisconsin-La Crosse found that "wall practice [is] neither a help nor a hindrance in juggling skill acquisition. Several [subjects] in the wall group remarked that they felt dependent upon the wall for optimal performance [after training this way]" (Catanzariti, 1998).

quickly so you can focus on catching—but that fast tempo means you'll be stressed out and rushed to make wild catches.

Try slowing down the rhythm of the throws. My challenge to jugglers who make errors in throwing too quickly: Try to make an error where you juggle too slowly, instead. Sometimes the proper tempo is far slower than beginner jugglers imagine, and they won't discover the appropriate rhythm unless they're told to make the opposite mistake intentionally.

Problem: Coming Down Too Quickly

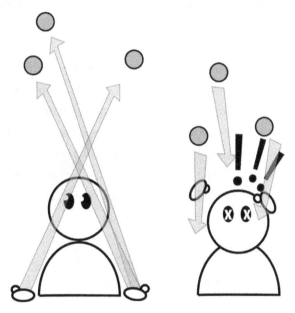

Three up, three down. The faster you throw, the faster they hit you.

When you throw things up in rapid succession, they fall back down in rapid succession. If you're feeling rushed, try slowing down the timing of your throws. Also, check to make sure that you're not reaching up to make catches. If you catch higher, you're effectively making your throws lower (that is, you're reducing the amount of time it takes for a throw to return to a hand). And remember the old juggling adage—if something hits you in the head, don't look up. *There's more coming.*

Problem: "I've Been Practicing for Hours, and Not Making Any Progress!"

Take a nap. No, really. Stop juggling and go to sleep. In 2016, a group of researchers from Tokyo's Waseda University conducted a study about the effects of sleep and napping on the process of learning three balls. They had two groups of learners—a nap group, and a no-nap group—who set out to learn to juggle. Both groups had hourlong training sessions, twice a day, facilitated by an instructional DVD.

The nap group took a 70-minute power-nap after training, and the no-nap group remained awake. A few hours after the napping group awoke, they had another training session. The group that napped enjoyed a vast improvement relative to the non-napping group, and this effect carried through to the next morning's training session. The researchers concluded that these results provide "...convincing justification for introducing nap periods into daily athletic training as an active method to improve performance, not just as a passive opportunity for recovery from fatigue" (Morita, Ogawa, & Uchida, 2016).

In other words: If you want to get better at juggling, take a nap after you train and the skills you're learning will gel more quickly.[11]

Problem: The Two-Ball Shuffle

A common problem for new jugglers is to fall into a strange two-ball shuffling pattern. In siteswap notation, this is known as "31". If you're making a throw from your dominant hand and simply handing the next

---

11 There is also evidence that using a form of virtual reality training is also an effective method of isolating subskills related to juggling—throw timing, rhythm, etc (Lammfromm & Gopher, 2011). Unless you've got easier access to VR technology than you do a bed, let's just stick with napping.

throw across, you should go back to the "Throw, Throw, Catch, Catch" and "Throw, Throw, Get Rid of It!" drills. Remember—in the three-ball cascade, all of the balls are thrown into the air!

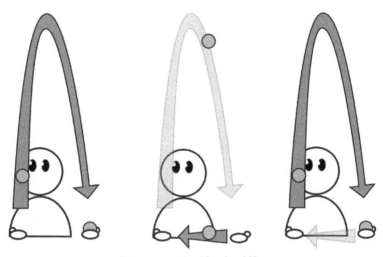

The two-ball shuffle.

GENERAL TRAINING TIPS

Before we begin, I'd like to offer some general advice for your juggling practice. Feel free to bend the corner of this page for quick reference later on—you'll probably want to come back as you progress through the book.

• It's better to practice for five minutes a day than one long session once a week.

• Be mindful of everything that's going on—ask yourself why something isn't working. Examine. Take notes.

• It's okay to follow your "natural syllabus"—you'll learn fastest if you're training something that interests you. If you find that fancy starts and finishes are more fun than training endurance one day, focus on that and you'll get more out of your session.

• It's important to train technique every time you practice, even if it's not the main focus of the day's session. Touching on it daily will help you achieve long-term success.

• Finish on a high note, with a trick or a sequence that you can do reliably.

• Be sure to warm up before you really dive into a session. This is both for injury prevention and also to make sure you don't develop bad form. (Head to Appendix E if you want some warm-up tips!)

• Make short-, medium-, and long-term goals and train accordingly. Write the goals down, along with general plans to get there. If your goal is to learn five balls, then your goals might be "learn to juggle three very high and accurately," "get twenty rounds of 5551," and "learn to balance a stick on my forehead for two minutes without moving my feet." Whatever your goals are, think about how to achieve them.

• There are three distinct forms of "practice" in juggling: *practice, training,* and *rehearsal. Practice* is when you arrive in the space with an open mind, trying new things while washed in a sense of play. *Practice* is great if you're looking to discover new tricks or generally have a fun session. *Training* is more goal-oriented—you're in the studio to solidify tricks and measure growth of your skills. *Rehearsal* is the final step—it's where you train sequences of tricks to get the "phrases" smooth and solid. This is done with an audience in mind.

• Take your time. It's more important to do things well than it is to do them quickly.

• Find other people to juggle with! The juggling community is large—it circles the globe! There's a good chance a juggling club meets in your city already. Hop online and try to find them!

• Post training clips on social media! It feels nice to get feedback from friends and jugglers from around the world. Take part in the community!

• Video your training sessions and compare your technique across time. Compare your technique with professionals and other people with online videos.

THREE BALLS: THROWS TO KNOW

We're about to elevate your three-ball juggling with a whole series of new tricks! Before we begin, let's go over a new concept.

Throws have names. These names are actually numbers. This is part of a counting system that's called *siteswap notation*.

The throw you've been practicing—that staple of the three-ball cascade, moving from one shoulder to the other with a peak around the top of the line of sight—is called a *3*. This is because it is in the air for three beats, but that's beyond the scope of this chapter.

If your curiosity is getting the better of you, skip on over to Appendix A. That chapter details siteswap notation in extensive detail. (For our purposes now, though, all you need to know is that numbers represent different throws.)

In this chapter about three ball juggling tricks, we'll add a handful of new throws that are represented with different numbers. These throws are *1, 2, 4,* and *5*.

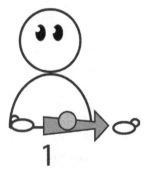

1 is a throw that goes directly from one hand to the other. It's like you're clapping your hands and you happen to pass a ball between the two. The force of the throw comes from the heel of the thumb pushing it across.

2 is a hand-hold or a very small throw. The ball does not change hands.

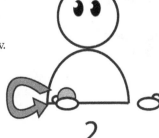

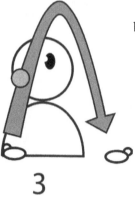

3

3—you know this one already! This is the basic throw in a three-ball cascade.

4 is a throw that goes straight up and down. It's taller than a 3 and stays on its same side. If the left hand throws it, that same left hand will catch it.

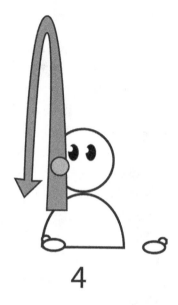

4

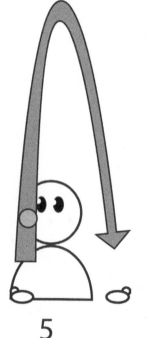

5

5 is the older brother of the 3. It's about twice as high as a 3 and crosses from one hand to the other.

...Are there profound mathematical implications to these numbers and throws? Yes, there are! The deeper implications are addressed at great length in Appendix A at the end of this book. For now, just treat these new numbered throws as vocabulary words and you'll be fine—when you're invited to throw a "4," make a vertical toss that stays in the same hand that peaks higher than a "3" would, and so on. Excited? Good! Turn the page and let's get started!

THREE-BALL JUGGLING: THE NEXT STEP

ONCE YOU'VE LEARNED to juggle three balls for 20 catches or so, you're probably itching to learn something new. Fear not! Here I show you the next steps in your juggling progression. Don't just pay attention to the trick here, pay attention to the progression we use to learn it.

441—Your First Siteswap
Or: How to Learn a New Siteswap

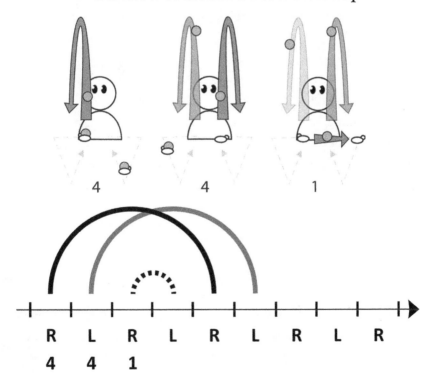

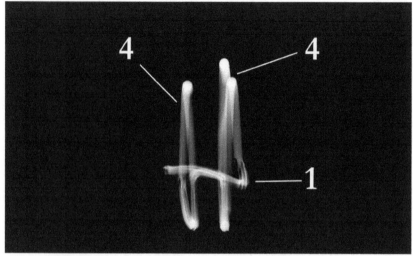

Siteswap 441. Notice the scoop of the 4s that extends below the horizontal line of the 1.

"Up, up, over." This is the first juggling pattern that was discovered through siteswap notation. 441 is an extremely important pattern to learn if you're interested in juggling four balls, but it's also quite pretty in its own right.

If you look at the siteswap—441—it only contains two different types of throws. Two 4s—throws which are vertical, returning to the hand that threw them, followed by a single 1—a hand-pass from one side to the other. When you first work on this, imagine the 1 being like clapping—one hand places the ball into the other. It's barely a throw at all and has virtually no time in the air whatsoever.

Drill: The Cold Start

Let's begin!

Start learning this pattern "cold"—that is, without any kind of lead-in throw. Numbers in a siteswap are like a computer code. A single number represents a single throw. When we start working with 441, we'll execute exactly three throws. A 4, a 4, and then a 1. Catch, catch, catch, and you're done.

The important thing at this point is to go slowly. Make the first throw. It should be higher than the 3 of the cascade pattern you've been practicing up until this point. Release the second throw just before the first throw reaches its peak. While those two balls are in the air, you throw the 1, which is a simple hand-pass from one side to the other.[12] When you first start, it's more important that you place good mental effort into the throws than it is that you catch them. (Remember? General to specific! We're shaping the pattern here. Think about making nice throws, think about the timing, and the catches will magically happen.)

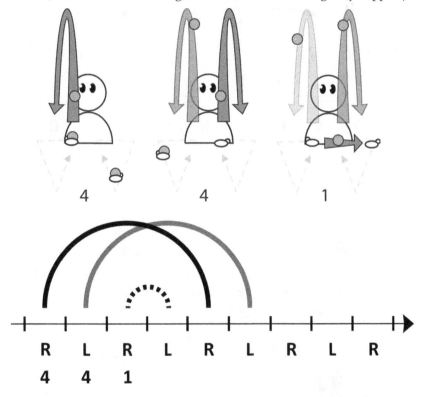

441 in isolation—make these three throws, then stop!

---

12 When you first start making this throw, you'll probably bring your hands together as though you are clapping. That's okay! With time, this hand-pass will likely turn into a throw. For now, do what feels good!

Drill: Back into Cascade

The next step is throwing 4413. All we're doing is adding a single throw—instead of stopping at three total throws, now we add a new one, our friend the 3, that same cascade throw that you've been working on since you started this book.

If you look carefully at the following ladder diagram, you'll notice that the 1 turns into the 3 that follows it. I tell my more visual learners that it's like setting a mousetrap—the 1 is pulling the wire backward and the 3 is releasing the spring.

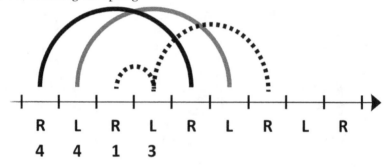

R	L	R	L	R	L	R	L	R
4	4	1	3					

4413—Notice the new throw made with the dotted line.

Just like the "throw, throw, get rid of it!" exercise when learning the three-ball cascade, we care more about the timing and execution of this new throw than we do a successful catch. The more you practice and push yourself, the faster this new throw will become exactly the same as a 3 in your three-ball cascade. Once it is, you're ready for the next step.

Drill: 441 Back into Three

Once you have successfully executed 4413, it's time to do the same exercise, only add an infinite number of 3s to our little computer program. That is to say, do a 441 from a cold start and then go back into a three-ball cascade.

When you can do this confidently several times in a row, it's time to move on to the next step.

Drill: Three into 441

In this exercise, we juggle a three-ball cascade. When we're feeling good and ready, we throw 441.

There will be a moment of panic. That's normal. This is a new thing! We're learning! Before you make your first 4 throw out of a cascade, however, I need to ask you a question.

Where does this 4 go?

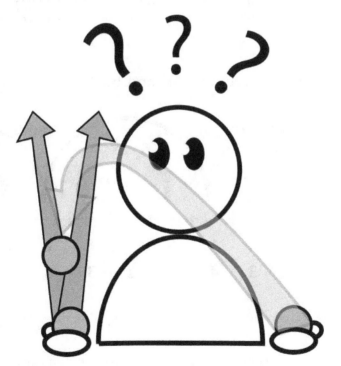

Where does the 4 go? Inside or outside of the descending 3?

A 4 is a vertical throw. However, there is a 3 descending into the hand that's about to throw it. And now you need to make a choice. Does this 4 go on the *inside* of the descending 3? Or does it go on the *outside*?

The most important thing for you to think about as you first work on this exercise is to always make the 4 on the inside of the incoming 3.

There's a reason for this. Remember our hand scoop? Keeping our throws to the inside allows us to maintain this hand-motion. If we throw to the outside, we need to change the direction of the hand scoop, which drastically impacts the efficiency of our movements. In the future, we will absolutely break this rule. For now, we're working on making good habits that will serve you as you progress through this book. The stronger your foundation, the more quickly you will progress.

That being said, give it a go. Juggle a three-ball cascade, throw a beautiful, tall 441 (with the 4s going higher than your 3s, of course,) and collect.

Drill: Three into 441 and back into Three

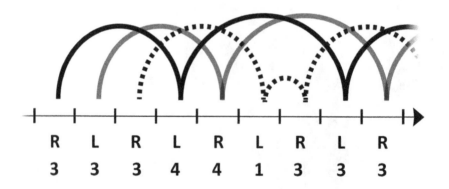

In this step, we combine both exercises. Juggle a three-ball cascade, throw a 441, then go back into a three-ball cascade.

Once you feel confident starting the 441 pattern with one side, start the 441 with the other hand. I'm not being mean (I swear!)—I'm just preparing you for the next step.

Drill: Repeating 441s

R	L	R	L	R	L	R	L	R
4	4	1	4	4	1			

You're now ready to run the pattern 441. This means that instead of the 1 turning into a 3 on the next beat, it turns into a 4. The pattern we're going to execute is 441441—doing the same pattern twice.

441 is not a "sided" pattern. That means that when we repeat it, the pattern switches sides. It's symmetrical. In the first 441, the 1 goes one way. In the second, it goes the opposite way.

Remember—after the first round of 441, we need to make sure we're starting the new throws on the *inside* of the incoming ball, just as we did when we went from a three-ball cascade into 441.

Applying this Process to Other Patterns

Let's repeat what we just did:

First, we learned how to do this new pattern in isolation—only throwing exactly the numbers that were on the page. In this case, it was three total throws: 4-4-1.

Then, we made a single new throw—we added a 3.

After that, we went from the new pattern back into our base pattern (in this case, it was the three ball cascade; for a four-ball siteswap, you'd do a four fountain).

Next, we went from the base pattern into the new pattern.

Then, finally, we went from the base pattern into the new pattern, and then back into the base pattern.

Why?

Training like this allows you to gain familiarity with the new throws in isolation. You don't need to worry about all of the throws and catches that will eventually surround them.

Adding a single throw of the base pattern after the new siteswap allows you to gain familiarity with the transition—going from the new thing back into the old thing.

As we enter fully into the base pattern in the following step, we are given the opportunity to notice the tempo of the balls as we re-enter the base pattern. This gives you additional information about the height of the throws—if there's a strange syncopation as the balls return to your hands, you know that something was too low or too high.

In the next step, we went from the base pattern into the new pattern. This allows you to examine the tempo from the opposite side. In this drill, you feel the metronome as you make the new throws—are you experiencing the same issues?

In the next step, you get to see how everything lines up. How is the timing? How are the throw heights? Does everything fit with the metronome?

Finally, we simply run the new pattern without the base pattern on either side. We know that it will be successful because we have examined all of the aspects of this new pattern in isolation, allowing errors to become salient.

This training method is all about "vocabulary building"—that is learning how new throws relate to one another against your internal metronome. In my experience, if you train new siteswaps this way, you will gain a much stronger foundation as a new juggler and progress much more quickly. You're establishing these new throw heights in your brain and body in a way that forces you to pay attention to small errors rather than simply throwing, dropping, and picking everything back up.

THREE-BALL SITESWAPS FOR BEGINNERS

These aren't in any particular order, so find a trick that sounds cool and get cracking! We'll start with three-ball siteswaps first and then get into other tricks.

When you begin working on these patterns, use the same method that we just used with 441. Start with the new pattern in isolation—each number is a simple bit of computer code that represents a single throw—start cold, juggle one cycle of the pattern, and stop cold. Then, begin the process of executing the pattern into and out of a three-ball cascade. Then, learn to repeat the new pattern.

Siteswaps not your thing? That's totally all right! This chapter and the following one—"Three-Ball Variations"—are your sandbox. If something looks like a fun thing to try, go for it! Follow your internal syllabus! The important thing to know, though, is that some of the siteswaps in this current chapter are important to understand and execute before you move along to the chapters on four- and five-ball juggling.

423

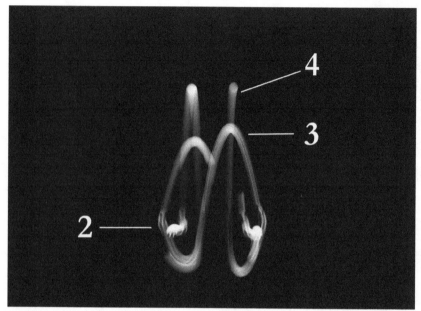

Above: 423 with inside 4s.

Below: 423 with outside/reverse 4s.

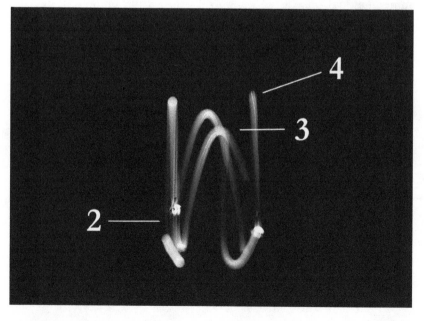

This W-shaped pattern is the building block of many juggling tricks.

When you first work on this, you probably won't be aware of the 2 at all, since it's simply a hand-hold where nothing happens. The pattern will have a strange, loping rhythm—right, right, left, left...

Later on, we'll take a look at identifying the 2. Even later than that, we'll learn how to create new tricks using 423 as the base pattern. (If you'd like to skip ahead and check that out, flip on over the chapter titled "The Shaky 2s").

Looking at the LED photos on the opposite page, you'll notice that they look different. The one on the bottom uses reverse throws—that is, the 4s are on the outside, with a scoop that travels from the inside to the outside. Experiment with both techniques!

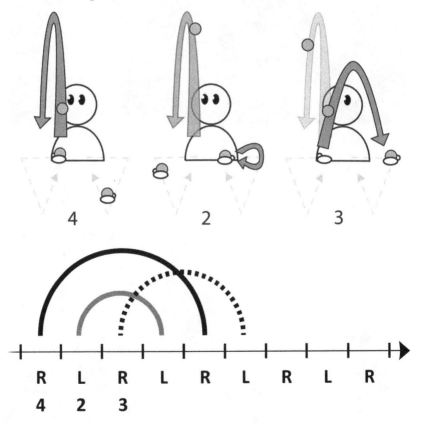

531

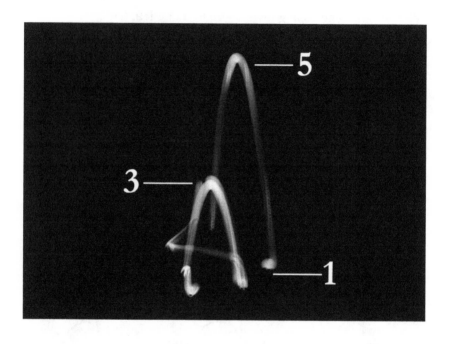

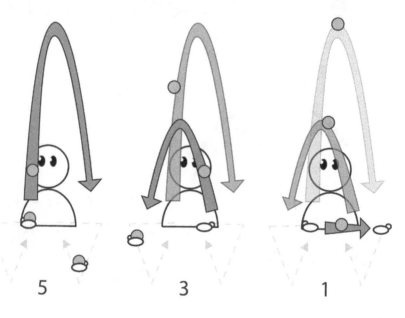

5   3   1

This is the first of the "tower patterns" that you'll learn. In 531, you throw all three balls at different heights, catching them in the reverse order.

When this trick is done perfectly, all three of the balls will peak in the air at the same time, creating a brief moment of suspense where they're all hanging in the air in a beautiful straight line. (Don't believe me? Check out the last frame of the cartoon on the opposite page!) When you eventually start working on the four- and five-ball versions of this trick (7531 and 97531, respectively), this effect will become more and more salient.

New jugglers often have an issue with this trick where the 5 is too low or the 3 is too high. When you start practicing this pattern, work on a single cycle entering and exiting the the three ball cascade. As you do this, pay attention to the rhythm as you re-enter the cascade. Is there a strange staccatto as you return to the base pattern? If there is, one of your throws isn't proportional.

Once you've mastered this pattern—running it for 10 or 20 cycles—try to do something interesting with the 1. Can you make that pass behind your back? Behind your neck? Under your leg?

This pattern looks quite ugly when it's done at first. How can you make it beautiful?

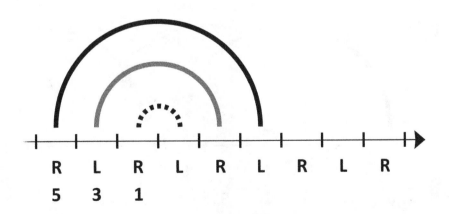

Shower: 51

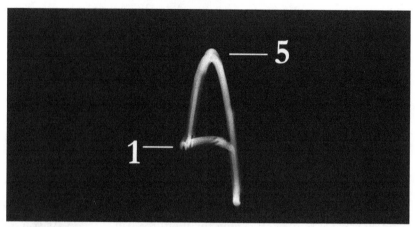

The three ball shower, or 51. Notice the "scoop"— appearing as a vertical line on the far right side—can be seen as the 5 is released.

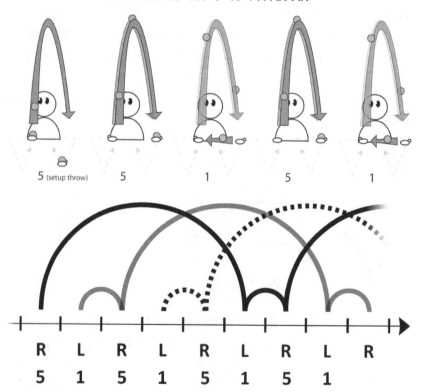

51 is commonly known as the three-ball shower. It's the pattern most jugglers attempt when they try to teach themselves to juggle three balls—and, in fact, it's a common pattern that's found in traditional juggling games around the world from antiquity until today.

It's important to remember that this is an asynchronous pattern, meaning that one hand throws a 5, then the opposite hand passes a ball across as a 1. It's possible to do the trick synchronously, but that turns it into (4x,2x).[13] For our purposes, you should learn the asynchronous version of the three ball shower first. After you've mastered the asynchronous three-ball shower, feel free to experiment with synchronous time.

The three-ball shower is an excited state siteswap, meaning that it needs a special set-up throw to transition into the pattern from the three ball cascade. To enter the pattern, you need to throw a 4. (So: 33333…4515151…) To exit, throw 23. This will feel like a pause in the pattern. In siteswap notation, these transition throws are separated with a vertical line: |. Formally, this full pattern would be written as "4| 51 |23".

When you first start working on it, though, work on the pattern from a cold start—that is, without trying to enter it from your base three-ball cascade. In order to do this, you need to start by throwing two 5s from the starting hand—you can see this in the cartoon, where the first 5 is marked as "set-up throw."

Remember to make the 5s nice and tall. We're working on precision rather than handspeed, after all! If you find that your pattern tends to speed up or collapse as you work on it, your 5s are probably getting too low. This is often due to muscle fatigue. Think about making each 5 slightly higher than the last and you'll trick your brain into making equal-height throws, counteracting your tired arms.

Box: (4,2x)*

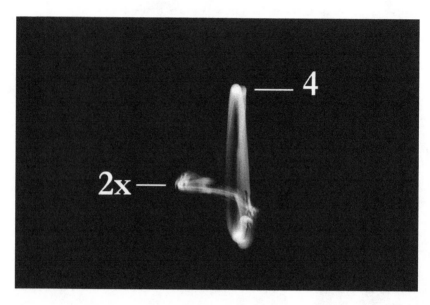

Above: One side of the box pattern
Below: The box pattern, repeated on both sides

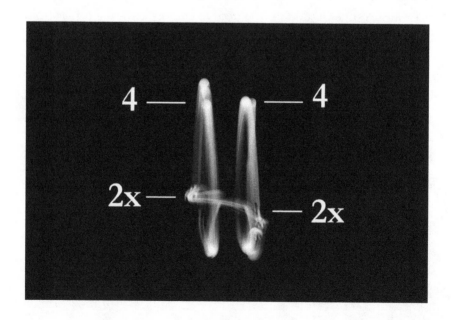

The box is a synchronous version of 423, and it's often the first synchronous pattern jugglers learn. The notation for synchronous patterns is a bit different than asynchronous patterns—please refer to Appendix A before working on this one!

The pattern is (4,2x)*—meaning that you throw a 4 at the same time as a 2x (the same hand-to-hand shuffle as a 1, but notated for synchronous time... if the notation is confusing, don't worry about it! Some of these concepts take a while to fully understand.)

When you start working on this pattern, drill it with two balls. First, you'll throw (4,2x). Both of these throws happen at the same time. The 4 goes up, and the 2x is caught underneath it. I like to think of this like a seesaw—a space opens up, and a ball is handed across underneath to fill the space.

When the 4 starts its descent, pass the 2x back underneath to your open hand. Practice this on both sides.

When you go to add the third ball, it's the exact same drill. If you find yourself rushing, your 4s are probably too low. Don't be afraid to push those throws up to slow down the metronome.

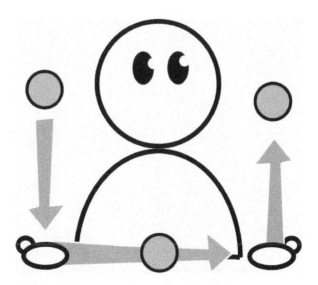

THREE-BALL VARIATIONS

Siteswap only describes how long it takes for an object to return to a hand—it doesn't say anything about where the ball actually travels. A 3 thrown behind the back is still a 3. A 4 throw under the leg is still a 4. A 5 that travels over the top of the pattern is still a 5. A rose by any other name would smell as sweet. In this section, we'll explore a few variations with three balls that go beyond the siteswap.

The big takeaway here is that there is more time in a juggling pattern than you might initially think. These variations are an exploration of different ways to throw and catch objects. The way you throw determines the amount of time it takes for a ball to return to your hand—sometimes we'll even do something else while we're waiting for that ball to return, too! (This concept will become especially salient in the chapter "The Shaky 2s.")

This list is by no means exhaustive—there are an infinite number of possible variations in juggling. Hopefully this chapter inspires you to invent some of your own!

If you're looking for a more complete guide to three-ball juggling variations, look no further than *Charlie Dancey's Encyclopaedia of Ball Juggling* by our friends at Butterfingers Press.

Reverse Throw

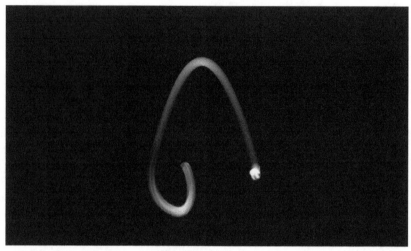

A reverse throw with a single ball. Notice how the scoop on the right starts from the inside and goes to the outside.

Reverse throws are made by changing the direction of your scoop. They're thrown from the outside position, peak at the corner of the throwing hand, and go down the outside of the pattern to the catching hand.

Remember the "mountains and rainbows" discussion from the chapter on learning the basic cascade? This is that rainbow throw!

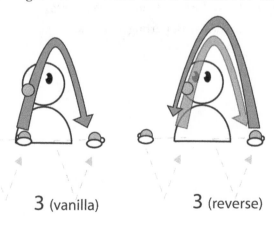

3 (vanilla)   3 (reverse)

Tennis

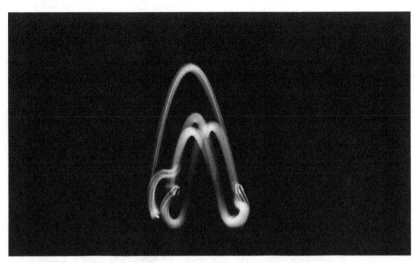

Three-ball tennis. One ball is thrown in reverse, traveling back and forth over the other two balls. The bottom two balls are manipulated with regular inside throws.

Three-ball tennis is a pretty trick, where a reverse throw is stuck in an orbit, being thrown over the top of the pattern. It's called "tennis" because the over-the-top throw looks like it's lobbed back and forth like the ball in a tennis match. The siteswap for this pattern is just 3 – though a ball is being thrown over the pattern, it's mostly a change of direction with very little change to the throw's height.

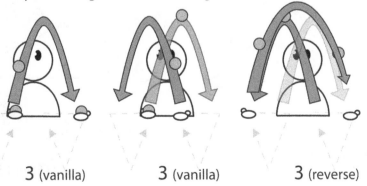

3 (vanilla)   3 (vanilla)   3 (reverse)

Half Shower

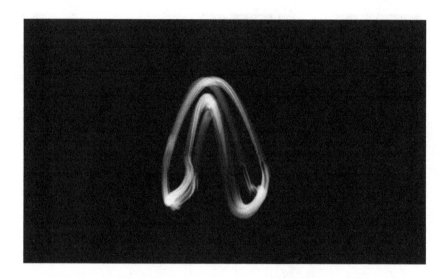

In a half shower, one hand makes all reverse throws and the other hand makes all normal inside throws. This shape has a triangle shape that's similar to the shower, but is still siteswap 3 because the bottom throws are tossed. not handed across..

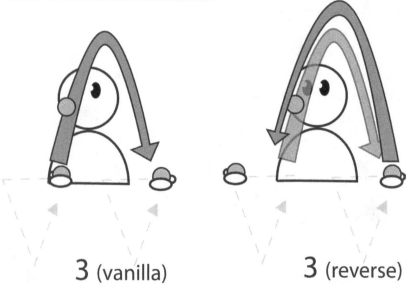

3 (vanilla)   3 (reverse)

Reverse Cascade

In the reverse cascade, all throws are thrown in reverse. This means that the balls all peak on their own side and land on the inside of the hand scoop.

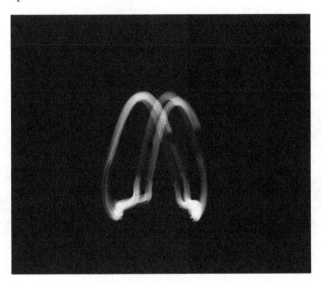

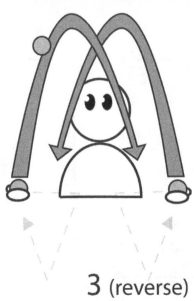

3 (reverse)

Columns

This pattern is also called "one up two up." It's siteswap (4,4)(4,0). Two balls go up and down together, and the other one is alone. Nothing changes hands in the basic version, but there are also some nice variations like (4,4)(4x,0)* where the solo ball travels from hand to hand.

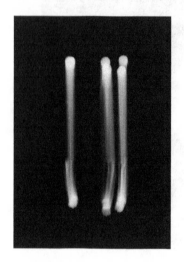 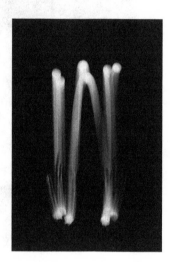

Left - (4,4)(4,0)
Right - (4,4)(4x,0)*

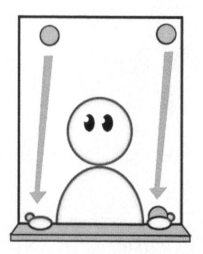 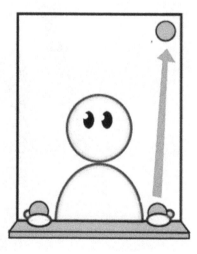

Yo-yo/Dumbwaiter

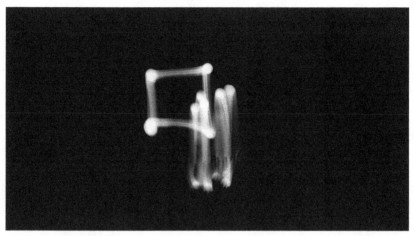

(4,2)—here, the 2 is held while the hand traces the outline of a square.

The Yo-yo and the Dumbwaiter are simple patterns but are often audience favorites. The siteswap here is 42 – that is, two balls juggled in one hand, with one ball held in the other.

The Yo-yo is a trick where the held ball moves up and down, mirroring the movement of one of the thrown balls while keeping an exact distance above it. If you move the held ball up and down below the throw ball, that trick is colloquially known as the Oy-oy.

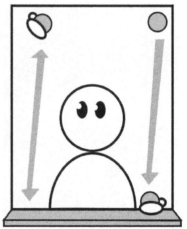

The Dumbwaiter

The Dumbwaiter is the same trick, but the held ball moves up and down alongside the thrown ball instead of above it.

While you juggle those two balls in your hand, you can move the held ball in a variety of ways, some with great effect! That's it!

Elbow Hits

The siteswap for a basic elbow hit is 42. A ball is thrown up and over to the opposite side. The opposite side's elbow taps the ball back to the hand that threw the ball. Since it returns to the hand that threw it, that throw is a 4. The side that makes the elbow tap is holding a ball, making that ball a 2.

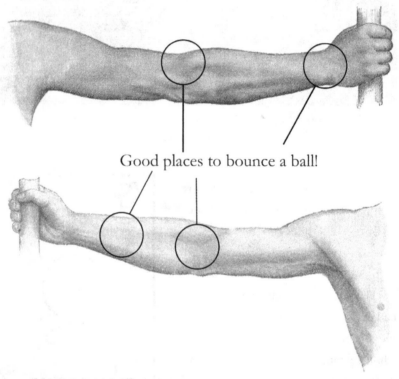

Good places to bounce a ball!

Above: Good places to bounce a ball. Adapted from "Gray's Anatomy plates 1231 & 1232" by Henry Gray, 1918 (https:// en.wikipedia.org/wiki/Upper_limb#/media/File:Gray1231. png)Public domain image.

Opposite page: The trajectory a ball follows when thrown with the right hand under the same and opposite legs. Adapted from Plate XXXIII of Osteographia by William Cheselden, 1733 (https:// www.nlm.nih.gov/exhibition/historicalanatomies/cheselden_ home.html). Public domain image.

Under the Leg

A throw under the leg is generally performed as a 3—so in a three-object cascade, there is no change in tempo.

When you first start working on under the leg throws, you have two options: Opposite leg or the same-side leg? Or, if you make the throw with your right hand, should you throw under your right leg or your left leg?

I find that it's easiest to learn this throw by throwing under the leg opposite from your throwing hand. This permits your arm a wider range of motion. Lift your leg up, reach across your body and underneath the crux of the knee, and you'll easily be able to make a beautiful throw to be caught by your opposite hand. Lift your left leg, throw the ball underneath that leg with your right hand, then make the catch with your left hand. Your wrist will just barely pass across the underside of the knee as you make the throw.

Throwing under the same leg takes a bit more physical effort, but it is easier to run continuous throws under the legs with this method. (A bonus: Running the pattern with all under-the-leg throws looks absolutely frantic. It's a real favorite for audiences, though it does take considerable stamina to master.)

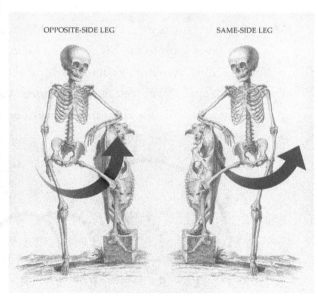

OPPOSITE-SIDE LEG   SAME-SIDE LEG

Eat the Apple (522)

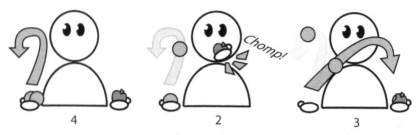

4   2   3

People have been juggling apples for millennia. In fact, the first recorded instance of an apple juggler was an Irish warrior named Cu-Chulainne, who could (allegedly) juggle nine apples that gleamed of silver back in the 11th century (Tain Bo Cuailnge, 2002)!

"Eat the apple" is a classic trick that can be done in any pattern with a 2 in it—usually a 423 or 522—where you take a chomp of the apple when it's in your hand on the 2 beat. (Remember to bite the apple, not a ball!)

If you're interested in learning this trick, remember to open your mouth before you bite. There are stories of people opening their mouths too slowly and smashing their teeth with the apple. The only thing worse than breaking a tooth is explaining how it happened to your dentist.

If you want to learn to eat three apples *all at the same time*, the pattern you use is 522. If you start with a right-handed 5, your left hand will simply hold its apple (2) as your right hand brings the apple it just caught up to be bitten (2). This one is a real race against time, so it might be best to start training it with a softer fruit.

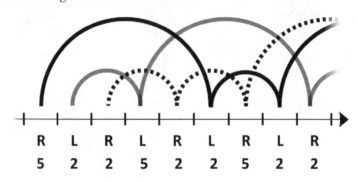

R	L	R	L	R	L	R	L	R
5	2	2	5	2	2	5	2	2

EXPLORING THE SPACE: THE SHAKY 2S

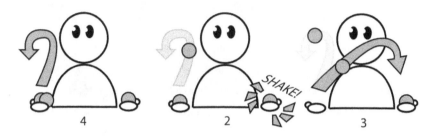

THIS IS ONE of my favorite drills for beginning three-ball jugglers. "The Shaky 2s" teaches you that there's more time in the pattern 423 than you realize and opens the door to thousands of exciting variations with an "active 2." An "active 2" is a 2-beat throw that doesn't just rest in the hand.

Though you might not feel it, there's a 2 in 423. This drill is learning to identify where that 2 happens, and marking it with a little shake. It may be helpful to think about the 2 in relation to the 4. When the 4 is in the air, the 2 is already taking place in the opposite hand.

At first, just try turning your wrist or making some other small motion to acknowledge the 2. As you gain confidence, you'll be able to make larger and larger movements.

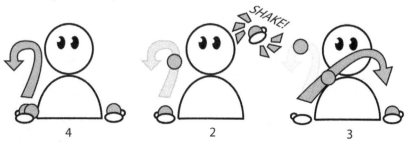

By discovering the location of this 2—and in learning to activate a motion during its beat—we open the door to a multitude of new three-ball juggling patterns.

A 2 by definition is a throw that returns to its hand exactly 2 beats after it's released. There's nothing else for that hand to do while its ball is in the air, which means that we can start playing with what that throw looks like (so long as it's back in its hand two beats later).

How many different 2s can you come up with? Here are a few ideas to get you going:

• Place the ball on a table and pick it back up.

• Swing your arm in a wide circle during the 2.

• Throw the ball over your shoulder, back to the same hand.

• Throw the ball to the top of your line of sight and catch it at its peak.

The pattern 423 is the building block of thousands of juggling patterns—all of which utilize the "extra" time that's afforded to us by the 2. By cultivating an awareness of timing with The Shaky Twos, you open up a world of possible juggling patterns.

MULTIPLEX STARTS

A MULTIPLEX THROW is a throw where multiple objects are released at the same time, from the same hand. They are controlled by two main factors: the line of the hand and the action of the wrist.

Think of the line that goes from your forearm through your hand, and up your middle finger. The vector that this line creates against the ground when the balls are released is an excellent predictor of how the balls will travel.

For example, if the throw is released with the line pointing slightly outward, with one ball farther away from you than the other, the balls will split diagonally away from you. If the balls are released with this arm-line perpendicular to the ground, the balls will travel upward and along the plane of your juggling "window."

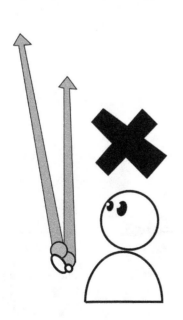
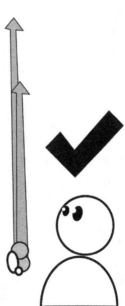

The more you flick your wrist, the wider the balls will split in the air. Learning to control the flick will permit you to make throws that have huge gaps in them, like an [84] or an [A4].[14]

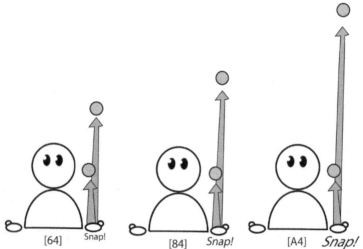

[64]   Snap!   [84]   Snap!   [A4]   *Snap!*

There are two main multiplex starts with three balls. In the first, ([84],6), one hand multiplexes two balls vertically. In the second, [654], one hand throws all three balls at one time—this throw can also be notated as ([86x4],0) in synchronous time. Though these patterns look totally different on paper, they're remarkably similar—if you were to take a photograph of these patterns in midair, you'll find that they both create the same "state" in the air. When the objects descend, you'll find that they land in such a way that you can begin juggling right away!

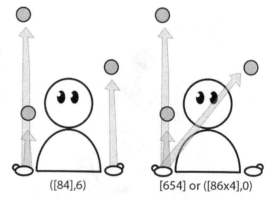

([84],6)   [654] or ([86x4],0)

---

14 Woah, what's that letter doing there? We switch to letters for throws taller than 9-beats high. If you'd like more information on this, head to Appendix A: "Siteswap: The Language of Juggling" on page 151!

TWO BALLS IN ONE HAND

For this chapter, we're handing the lesson to Benjamin Domask-Ruh. Benjamin is an amazing juggler and performer, who teaches this concept better than anyone else I know. Take it away, Benjamin!

Hold two balls in your hand, situated so that one ball is resting on your palm and secured by your ring and pinky fingers while the other is held primarily in the remaining fingers (thumb, pointer, and middle).

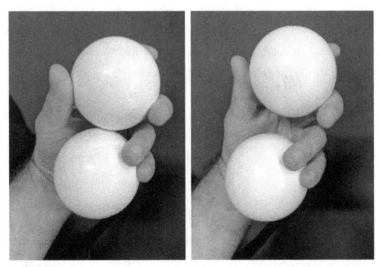

Hold two balls in one hand like this—the balls are gripped in a single hand, with groups of fingers holding each ball so they can be controlled independently of one another. These two images are of the same hand, gripping the balls in the same way. In the left image, the fingers are curled and the palm is contracted. In the right image, the fingers and palm are more extended.

This is our standard two-ball grip. It's the same as holding two balls in one hand to start a three-ball cascade.

As you stand in your good juggling stance of feet shoulder-width apart, knees slightly bent, and your weight securely over your heels, you must visualize a point above your shoulder. Let us assume you are using your right hand: Visualize the space above the right shoulder. A good practical height is to raise your arm straight upward as if you were asking a question in elementary school or reaching for an object on the top of the shelf. See the height your hand is raised to and understand this will be the proper height to start at for your body.[15]

The first ball thrown (Ball 1) is lofted upward with our scooping motion toward our visualized point. It will be higher than the normal (3) throw we have practiced with one ball and two hands. Another difference is that this ball will return to the same hand on the same side of the body instead of crossing our body to the opposite hand. Thinking back to our siteswap knowledge, we can identify this throw as a 4!

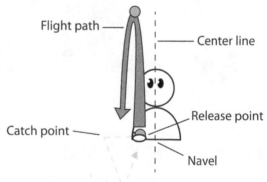

---

15 Credit where credit is due: I learned this tip from juggling coach Richard Kennison.

The proper path of this throw follows a tall, skinny oval shape coming from inside our shoulder (released near our navel) and returns outside of our shoulder (caught near our corresponding hip).

Practice throwing and catching Ball 1 while holding a second ball as stated above, so you will be throwing and catching the same ball from the fingers.

Once you have succeeded in throwing Ball 1 to the proper height and catching it 10 times in a row without dropping, it's time to attempt the second throw.

After we have thrown Ball 1, Ball 2 will be resting in your palm, anxiously awaiting to be thrown. As Ball 1 leaves the hand, the thumb, pointer, and middle finger close around Ball 2, and the hand is brought down again. The hand scoops and releases Ball 2 just as Ball 1 reaches its apex (our visualized point) and begins to descend back to our hand.

Catch Ball 1 as practiced and watch as Ball 2 comes down on the same path. The proper place to catch Ball 2 at this point will be in the fingers where Ball 1 started.[16]

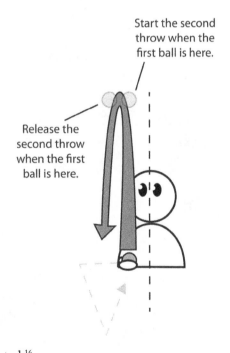

Start the second throw when the first ball is here.

Release the second throw when the first ball is here.

---

16 NOTE: As we begin to juggle two balls in one hand, it is not necessary to remember which ball is which. We have numbered the balls at this point to make it easier to comprehend.

Again, repeat this 10 times without dropping.

After you have found success, it is time for the third throw! As Ball 2 comes down and Ball 1 is caught in your hand, continue the slightly circular path your hand is automatically making by throwing inside your shoulder near the navel and catching outside near your hip. Find your hand back near your navel in an upward motion and release Ball 1, again aiming for the visualized point above your head. Catch Ball 2 as it comes down in your palm. Feel free to close all your fingers around Ball 2 until Ball 1 returns on the downward path and is caught by the fingers.

To continue juggling two balls in one hand, simply continue throwing and catching in this inward to outward motion jugglers call a fountain.

Remember to work on both hands slowly and equally. A balanced juggler is a true juggler!

PRO TIP: This is also the basis for juggling four balls! When we juggle four objects in their basic pattern, we juggle two balls in each hand at the same time.

LEARNING TO BALANCE

THIS CHAPTER IS AN INTRODUCTION to balancing objects on your face and learning your "center line." In a later chapter, we'll add the concept of "split-brain" combination tricks—specifically, the act of balancing an object while juggling simultaneously. To accomplish that feat, you rely on both active focus as well as your "lizard brain" to achieve an act of coordination.

...but don't just take my word for it. Here's what Paul Cinquevalli, arguably the greatest juggler who ever lived, had to say about balancing and juggling:[17]

> *Perhaps the hardest thing a juggler must learn to do is to see things without looking at them. This may seem a paradoxical statement, but it is, nevertheless, true. For example, when I am balancing a glass on straw on my forehead, and juggling five hats at the same time I never look at the hats; if I did so for even the hundredth part of a second the glass and straws would collapse, but I know instinctively the position of the hats, and can catch them and juggle with them just as easily as if I were actually looking at them.*
>
> *But it takes years of practice to acquire what I can only call this sort of double sight.*

- Paul Cinquevalli, "How to Succeed as a Juggler" (Cinquevalli, *How to Succeed as a Juggler*, 1909)

---

17 If you'd like to learn more about Paul Cinquevalli and his profound impact on the art of juggling, check out Modern Vaudeville Press' title *Juggling: From Antiquity to the Middle Ages*. The final chapters of this book address his impact on the English language—the first recorded use of "juggling" in the vernacular as an explicit reference to "throwing and catching objects using skill acquired through practice" was in reference to him and his work!

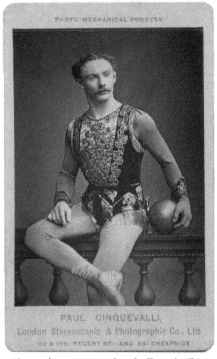

A promotional postcard of Paul Cinquevalli, circa 1890. From the author's own collection.

Learning to balance an object is an important part of developing your basic technique. When your body learns where its center line is, you will have a fundamentally better understanding of where to place objects in the air. Balancing objects is an extremely valuable tool when it comes to evaluating the crossing point of objects in the air and establishing better body posture when juggling. Learning to balance while juggling also helps you move some of your skills from "explicit knowledge and execution" phase (where your brain knows how to do something with conscious thought) to "implicit knowledge and execution" phase (where your body knows how to do something without conscious input from your brain).

This concept goes in hand with the famous psychologist Buch's "Four Stages of Competence": unconscious incompetence, conscious incompetence, conscious competence, and unconscious competence.

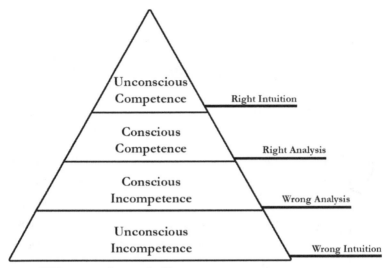

Hierarchy of Competence

The general idea (as it pertains to juggling) is that when you first work on a skill, you do not understand how to do it, nor do you understand the reasons why it's not working (unconscious incompetence). As your training progresses, you begin to understand how the trick works but still struggle to execute it (conscious incompetence). Further along, you begin to achieve success with serious concentration (conscious competence), and you eventually develop the skill to a degree of innate fluency (unconscious competence).

Our goal here is to get you to understand what you're doing, how to make it work, and get that information through your brain and into your body so you achieve success without even thinking about it.

If it offers any perspective, Anthony Gatto (or so the story goes) started his juggling training at the age of four or five in his father's tobacco shop. Before he started toss juggling, his father would throw a rubber ball to Anthony, and he'd bounce it back with his forehead. Anthony also learned how to balance objects as short as a teaspoon before he began learning to keep three balls in the air.

And, uh, Gatto turned out to be pretty good.[18]

Vocabulary

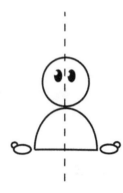

Center line: This is the central line within your body where balance is held. It's the same line that you rely on to balance on two feet when you're standing still. Here, we're extending that line up through an object. Just as you use your body's input to balance yourself upright, you're using your body's input to balance an object on your body.

Center of gravity: While the line of a balance runs through the object, the center of gravity is a single point. An object with a high center of gravity will be easier to balance than an object with a low center of gravity, as it's easier to read.

Juggling clubs[19] have a center of gravity in the bulb, about two thirds up the length of the club from the handle's knob. A wooden dowel

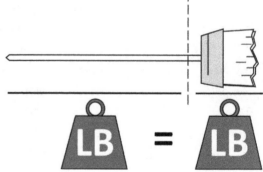

---

18 Read: The best technical juggler of modern times, even though he never learned to undestand siteswap notation!

19 Club juggling is beyond the scope of this book, but if you plan on picking up a set, this is good information to know!

has a center of gravity halfway along its length. A broom (pictured) has a center of gravity much closer to the bristles.

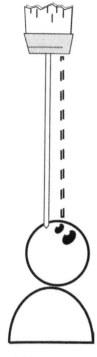

Reading: Reading an object refers to your ability to predict the way that it moves. In a balance, we read the movement of the object by sight and by its point of contact on the body. Objects are easiest to read when you look at their topmost point. (That's how you'll be learning, too!)

Picture plane: The picture plane is the two-dimensional representation of what's going on. When we talk about throwing an object so that it passes the top of the balance in our picture plane, that refers to the object appearing to go higher than the object we are balancing. Depending on where you balance the object (chin, nose, or forehead) and the angle of your neck, the thrown object may or may not actually travel higher than the top of the balance.

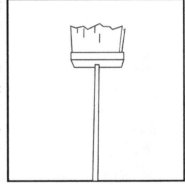

Let's Begin with a Balance

When you were a child, you may have experimented with balancing a broomstick on your hand. If you looked at the base of the broomstick, you had to run around to keep the object in precarious balance. When you looked at the top of the broomstick, you achieved control. Our first exercise is the same, though instead of a broomstick we'll use a 3' long, ½" diameter wooden dowel. And instead of your hand, we'll use your face. (But… on which part of your face?)

...Of course, there are more than just three. For the purpose of these initial exercises, we're talk about your chin, your nose, and your forehead.

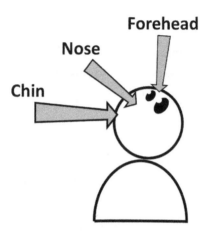

Chin

Pros: Easy to balance here; lots of nerve endings. In a comedy presentation, you can play up how difficult it is to talk at the same time. Your jaw is mobile, and when you have a solid balance here, you can use those muscles to make small corrections.

Cons: If you're a human with facial hair, you'll have to shave a ½" diameter circle at minimum. Stubble and hair can be slippery!

Nose

Pros: The ridge where your bone meets your cartilage is a massively sensitive area. You can "read" the balance very well here. It's also funny.

Cons: Different people have differently shaped noses: your mileage may vary with this balance. It's hard to place a club into a balance onto your nose out of a juggle. If you train the nose balance, get ready to poke yourself in the eye whenever you practice.

Forehead

Pros: In a workshop with Steven Ragatz, he insisted that this was the most dramatic way to balance an object. I agree. It also opens up your field of vision much wider.

Cons: This balance point requires you to flip your perception – since the balance occurs behind your eyes, toward the top of your picture plane, many people find this to be a huge challenge.

Which one should I pick?

You'll naturally find one balance point easier than the others. Use that little boost when you start training. The drills that follow train your mind—these skills will all transfer to other balance points.

Dowel Drills

This drill is simple and it also sucks. But it's the only way to build a solid foundation with balance. I first learned it from Richard Kennison but have heard it attributed to many different coaches as well. The earliest reference I've heard regarding this technique is by German juggling historian Karl Heinz-Ziethen.

A 3' dowel is balanced on the point of your choosing. Once it's placed in a balance, a two-minute timer is set. Once you can successfully balance the dowel for two minutes without moving your feet, you cut two inches from the length of the dowel. Rinse and repeat until the dowel is 10" in length.

Save these notches. Keep them on your desk at work. Paint them gold. Turn them into a bohemian necklace. These are your trophies. These are your measure of self-worth for the weeks and months you work on this drill.

Keep working on these endurance drills as you progress with the ball-juggling exercises in this book. You'll find them to be helpful as you carry on. I've included a series of drills to get you juggling while maintaining a balance toward the end of the book as well. Have fun!

One final big note: Be sure to check in with yourself! If you feel like your neck hurts, take a break! Watch out for a "crunchy" feeling in your spine and neck. There's no need to suffer. Crunchy feelings can be an indication of injury, as well... Stretch and be kind to yourself!

Four Balls: Throws to Know

Juggling four balls is "just" juggling two balls in each hand, at the same time.

Haven't tried it yet? Go for it. Two balls, one hand, siteswap 40. If you've been honest with your practice in 441 and 423, this should be a fairly quick pattern to learn. Be sure to juggle with a good, horizontal scoop. Many people face issues with a front-to-back "catapult" style scoop when they first attempt two in one hand. This can force you to walk backward and forward as you toss, as your scoop can project the ball in the axis perpendicular to your body rather than parallel to the line of your shoulders. A scoop that's in-plane with your shoulder—parallel to the "window"—makes for a relaxed posture with no front-to-back movement.

In this chapter, we'll meet the throws 6, 7, and 9. (...But don't forget about our friends 1, 2, 3, 4, and 5!)

6 is a 4's older brother. It's a vertical throw that's very tall.

7 is similar to a 3 or a 5. It still reaches across to the line of the opposite shoulder, but it's a full two beats taller than a 5.

9 is an extremely tall crossing throw. Just like a 5 or a 7, but yet another two beats higher than a 7.

Take a look at the diagram on the next page to see how these new throws compare to one another!

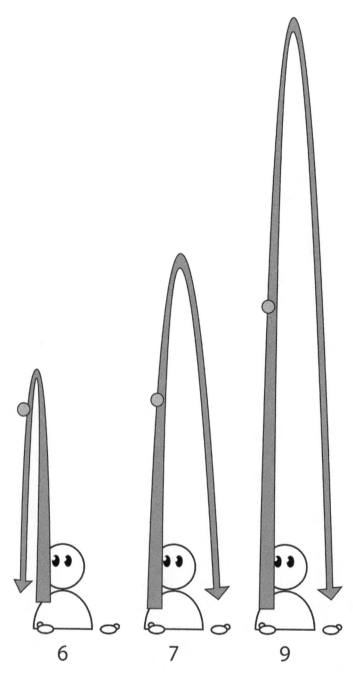

Throws to know when working on four balls.

LEARNING FOUR BALLS

FOUR-BALL JUGGLING is a representation of mastery with three balls. I'd recommend against working on four until you can proficiently run the three-ball pattern 441 for 10 cycles back to back.

The basic pattern for four balls is called the fountain. That's where you only juggle the siteswap 4—essentially "just" juggling two balls in either hand at the same time. This is exactly as we learned in the chapter "Two Balls in One Hand," where two balls are assigned to one hand and never cross the center line.

This can be accomplished either asynchronously (both hands throwing independently of each other, on their own beats) or synchronously ("bundling" pairs of throws with the hands throwing at the same time). This will be discussed in depth in Appendix A, but know that the asynchronous version of the fountain would be written down as "4" and the synchronous version of the fountain would be written down as "(4,4)." It is good practice to experiment with both synchronous and asynchronous fountains when you first begin practicing four-ball juggling.

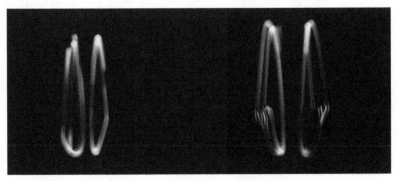

Left—Four balls asynch
Right—Four balls synch

The Most Common Error in Four-Ball Juggling

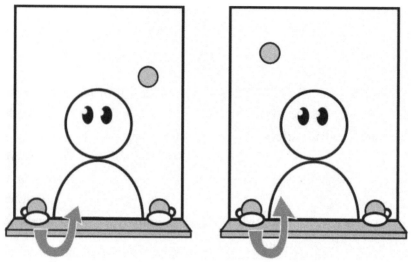

Left: the scoop for a 3-beat throw
Right: the scoop for a 4-beat throw
(Scoops exaggerated for clarity.)

When jugglers first start working on four balls despite having a proficiency with the three ball pattern 441—they often find that **the pattern collapses inwards on itself**. This has to do with the scoop and the timing of the ball's release in the scoop.

Since a 3 crosses and a 4 stays on the same side, they have different points of release. A 3 is released early in the hand's scooping circle, and the 4 is released slightly later. If the 4 is released too early in the hand's scoop, the 4-beat throws will drift inward, towards the center line.

If you are able to run the pattern 441 without moving your feet and without your body twisting or straining to make catches, you will likely avoid this common mistake!

Siteswaps with Four Balls

5551

5551 is a "sided" pattern—this means that when you run it for multiple rotations, it doesn't flip directions. If you start with your right hand, your right hand will always be throwing 5s and your left hand will always be doing the 5 and the 1. If we want to have this pattern flip directions, we need to add a 4.

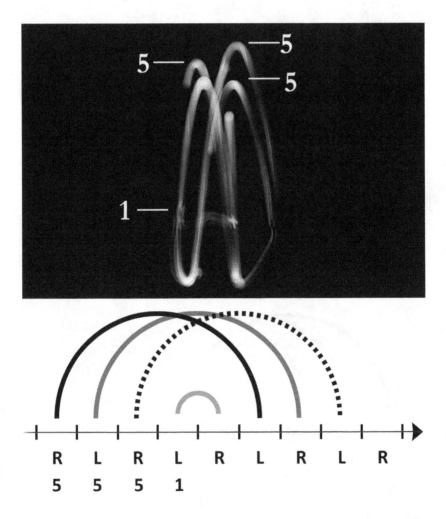

55514

55514 is the same pattern as 5551, just with a 4 added to it. This makes the pattern flip directions, since it changes the pattern's period (number of throws) from four to five.

This pattern is the gold standard for learning to juggle five balls. More on that in the five-ball chapter!

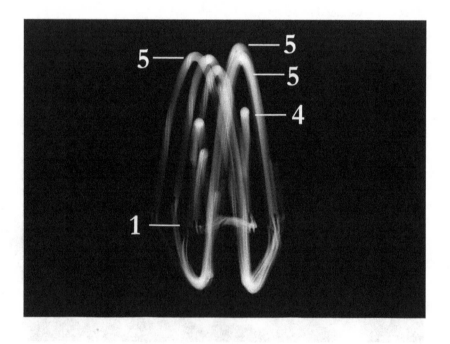

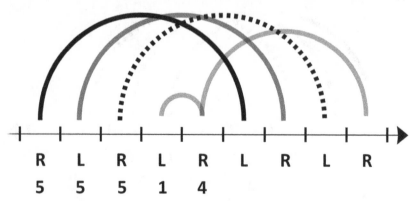

7441

"Chuck one high, then do 441!" If you're having a hard time with this pattern, you're probably making the 7 too low, the 4s too high, or a combination of the two. When you're getting ready for the high throw, sometimes the brain likes to tell the arms to make the rest of the throws higher, too. Focus on making the 7 nice and tall while maintaining 4s the same height as your fountain.

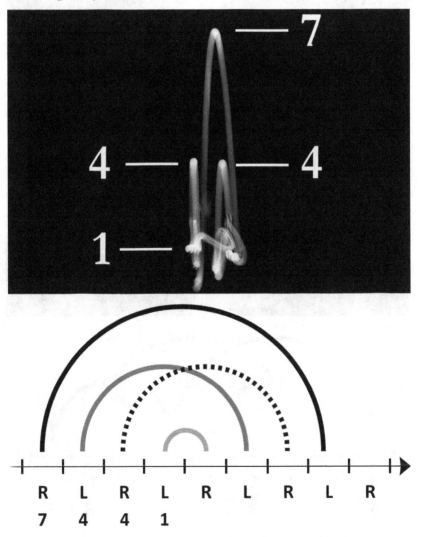

53

This is the half shower with four balls, usually executed with a reverse 5. This is a pretty, asymmetrical pattern, sometimes called "Popcorn."

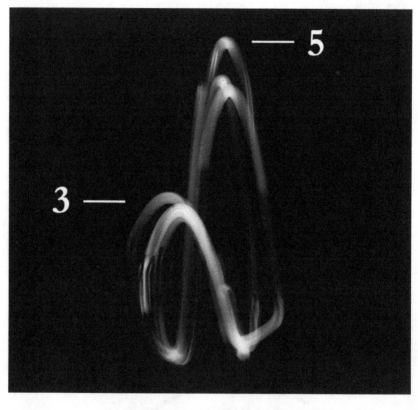

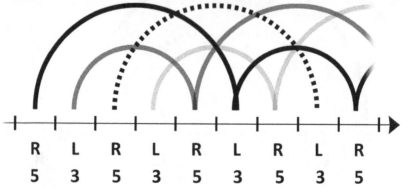

534

This pattern is in the same family as 423. It's a well-known standard in club juggling which lends itself nicely to interesting variations with balls as well!

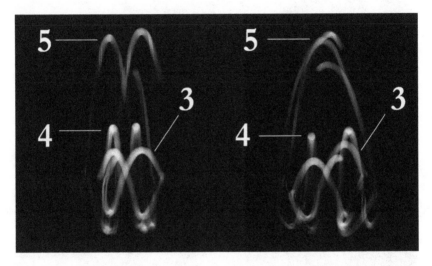

Left: 534 with vanilla 5s.
Right: 534 with reverse 5s.

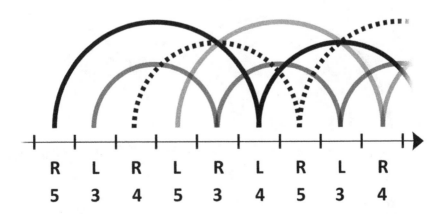

642

This is a "tower" pattern, where balls line up in midair. This pattern has a bit of a funny feeling, since it's only a period-three siteswap (only three throws) and one of them is a 2. Find that moment of suspension!

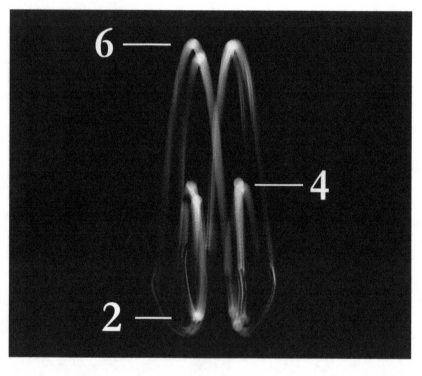

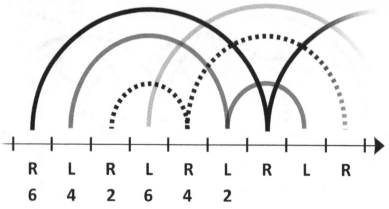

7531

This is the four-ball version of three's 531. This is a "tower pattern," where the balls all magically line up in the air and return back to your hands in reverse order. When you get it perfectly, it's magical!

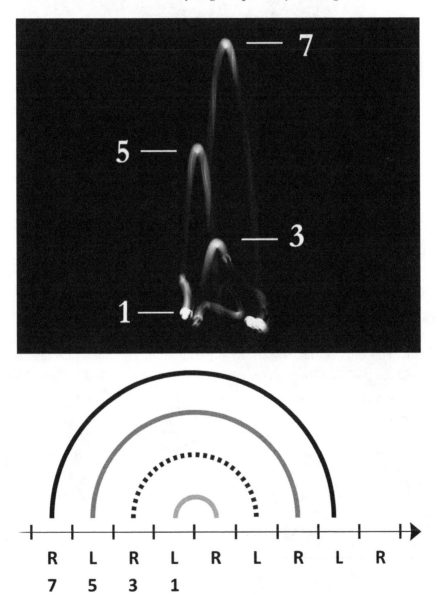

71

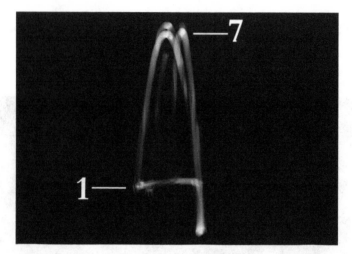

71 is the siteswap name for the four-ball shower—that classic triangle shape that so many people try to learn to juggle with. One hand makes tall throws and the other hand shuffles balls across so they can be thrown up again. As with 51—the three-ball shower—you may feel that the pattern collapses on you after a while. That's probably just fatigue. To combat this, think about making each 7 throw slightly higher than the one before it.

As with the three-ball shower, this is an "excited" pattern, meaning that you can't seamlessly transition into it from the four ball fountain without a setup throw. To enter the four shower, you'll need to throw 56 to enter the pattern. (So: 44444…567171717171….) To exit the pattern, you simply throw 42.

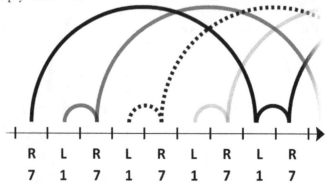

9151

This is a high-low variation of the four-ball shower, also known as a "double-headed shower."

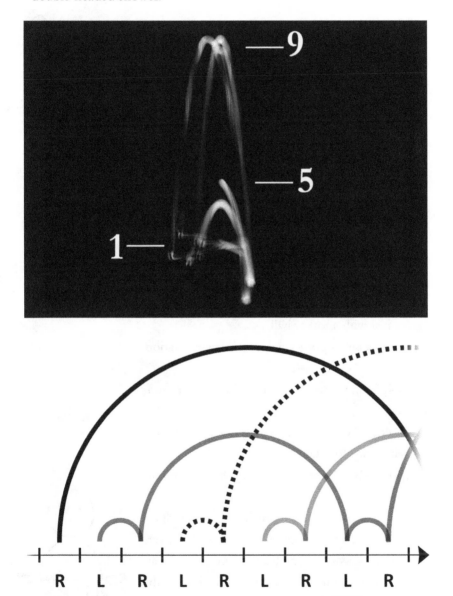

R	L	R	L	R	L	R	L	R
9	1	5	1	9	1	5	1	9

Multiplex Starts with Four Balls

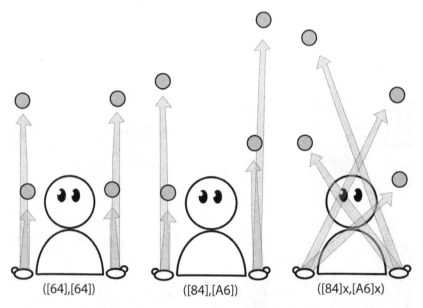

([64],[64])   ([84],[A6])   ([84]x,[A6]x)

There are a number of fancy starts with four balls that allow you to do different things. Here, we use the same technique as the three-ball multiplex starts, just with another ball.

To get a better grasp on this weird new notation, flip over to Appendix A!

([84],[A6]) : A way to get into the asynchronous fountain.

([84x],[A6x]]) : A fancy way to get into the asynchronous fountain.

([64],[64]) – A way to get into a synchronous fountain

Or how about the synchronous multiplex ([42],[86]x) as a way to get into a four-ball shower? This throw gets all of the balls to line up in the air then fall one by one into the hand that shuffles the bottom of the shower across.

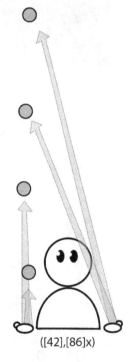

([42],[86]x)

ANYTHING CAN BE A HAND: APPLYING SITESWAP

SITESWAP NOTATION TELLS US about the number of beats—the amount of time—it takes for a thrown ball to be caught.

A 5 takes five beats to be caught after being thrown.
A 3 takes three beats to be caught after being thrown.
A 1 takes one beat to be caught after being thrown.

There's no rule that says that objects have to go in the air when leaving the hand, nor does it say where in space they have to travel (that's the same concept that tells us that complicated patterns like Mills Mess are just a bunch of 3s strung together!) The only thing that siteswap tells us is the amount of time it takes for an object to return to a hand. Remember, siteswap value does not always mean throw height!

So, what can we do with this information?

Instead of throwing a ball up into the air, we can do something else with it. Instead of throwing an 8, for example, we could place it on a table and pick it up eight beats later. Instead of throwing a 3, we could place the ball on top of our head and let it roll down and fall into the opposite hand. The longer a ball stays trapped or placed, the "higher" the throw. Since siteswap values only represent time, these are perfectly valid things to do.

This means that we can make old patterns look new! They're now denser, more compact, more dynamic and (some would argue) fresher!

Experiment with different places to put an object instead of throwing it. Here are a few examples to get you started:

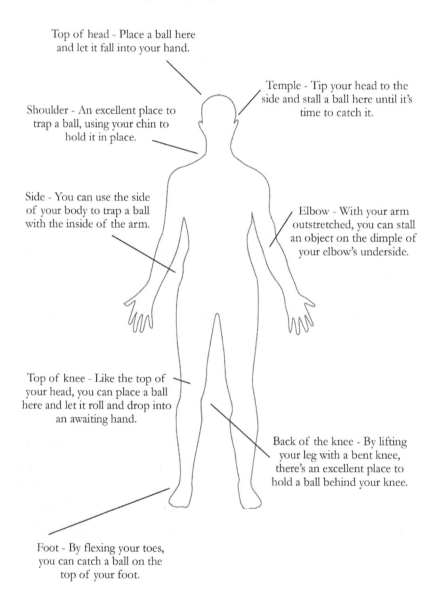

Top of head - Place a ball here and let it fall into your hand.

Temple - Tip your head to the side and stall a ball here until it's time to catch it.

Shoulder - An excellent place to trap a ball, using your chin to hold it in place.

Side - You can use the side of your body to trap a ball with the inside of the arm.

Elbow - With your arm outstretched, you can stall an object on the dimple of your elbow's underside.

Top of knee - Like the top of your head, you can place a ball here and let it roll and drop into an awaiting hand.

Back of the knee - By lifting your leg with a bent knee, there's an excellent place to hold a ball behind your knee.

Foot - By flexing your toes, you can catch a ball on the top of your foot.

Experiment with placing objects in these different places—or invent some of your own new places to stall an object!

Once you start to feel comfortable, try incorporating some of these new ideas within a juggling pattern. Use the siteswaps listed below. Traps, placements, and stalls are marked in bold. Experiment with elbow traps, foot catches, and other placements—put the ball anywhere!

The siteswaps below do not represent an exhaustive list of possibilities. If you have an idea for something that isn't on this list, go for it!

Three Balls

Try the following siteswaps, placing the **bold** number(s) somewhere instead of throwing it.

441

441

441

4**2**3

4**2**3

42**3**

(**4**,2x)*

51

531

5**2**2

52**2**

Four Balls

(**4**,4)

(8,2x)(**4**,2x)*

633

JUGGLING AND BALANCING/
BALANCING AND JUGGLING

100% of your focus, 100% of the time

HERE'S THE BIG SECRET—the hurdle that makes many beginning balancers stumble. When you're working on these drills, 100% of your focus is always on the balance. There's no quick glance to look at a ball to help catch it. There's no splitting your attention—not even 1% of it —to the juggling pattern. You focus on the balance, and let your lizard brain take care of the rest.

This chapter serves as a welcome relief to the army of diligent jugglers who have been working on their siteswaps up through this point. Although juggling with a balance is a fancy trick on its own, the following drills serve as a way to experiment and see how much of the material you've been working on to this point has "soaked in" to your body and is immediately accessible while focusing on another task. I like to refer to these drills as "brain-split" activities for this reason—what can you do while you're actively engaged with a balance on your face?

You're welcome to start playing with these drills before you have finished your dowel training to get a taste of it, but it will be a serious challenge.

Wavy Arms

With a club balanced on your face, raise your hands over your head and flail them wildly. Maintain focus on the club at all times.

This drill is good for two things—first, it introduces movement to your field of vision. If you look away from the club (even for a second!), it will fall. Don't get distracted! Second, raising your hands over your head will reduce your range of corrective motion. This makes maintaining the balance harder.

Throw and Catch

Balance a club on your face, then throw and catch a ball. Throw the ball as a 4, so it doesn't cross the line of the balance. Try to do this 10 times in a row with one hand, then 10 times in a row with the opposite hand.

To make it more difficult, try throwing a 6 or an 8. These higher throws should pass the top of the club in your picture plane. You'll likely find this to be disorienting.

This drill tests your focus, helping you realize that at no point are you ever allowed to lose focus on balance.

Down and Up

Balance a club on your face. Slowly sit down, then lie down on the ground. Can you get the back of your head to touch the floor without losing the balance? Stand back up while maintaining balance.

This drill is a nice measure of your proficiency with a balance and a nice way to see how small you can make your corrective movements.

The Reading Test

No balance involved with this one: Juggle three clubs while looking up at the ceiling. Trace the lines of the ceiling with your eyes. If there were a book on the ceiling, you could read it out loud. You'd be able to pass a reading comprehension test. This drill is to help you learn to trust your lizard brain. See? You don't have to think to be able to juggle!

The Face Cascade

This is a drill with three clubs. Balance a club on your forehead. Once you have control over the balance, hold another club and lower it onto your nose. When the nose club makes contact with your skin, shift your focus away from the forehead club, allowing it to drop while you maintain the new balance on your nose. When you have control over that club, place a club onto your chin. Again, once it makes contact with your skin, your focus will switch to the new balance, and the old balance will fall. From the chin, work your way back up, to the nose and then the forehead.

Do this drill with alternate hands (so, right to forehead, left to nose, right to chin, left to nose, right to forehead, etc).

This drill helps establish the rule of "100% focus on the balance at all times." It also helps you maintain balance with movement happening in your peripheral vision.

Place into a Balance

Juggle three clubs, and place one on your face in a balance. The final catch happens after you place the club in a balance. Think about making the last throw slightly higher than normal, so you have extra time to make the catch after you place into a balance.

This drill helps you shift focus—the second a club is placed into a balance, 100% of your focus shifts to that. The final catch is made by your lizard brain and is spotted passively with your peripheral vision.

Adding the Juggle

Once you've mastered the "throw and catch" drill, it's time to start adding a three-club juggle. (You can learn this with balls if you'd prefer, but that's much more challenging.)

You'll begin just as you learned to juggle for the first time—starting off with a two-club "throw, throw, catch, catch."

When you do this drill, make sure that the knobs are crossing into the bottom of your picture plane—into your peripheral vision—as they travel into their respective corners. We're not juggling blind; we're allowing our lizard brain to interpret the club's trajectory based on that small bit of input.

As always, you're allowed to drop the juggle, not the balance. 100% of your focus on the balance at all times!

FAQ

Where do I hold my hands?

Hands are funny things. Especially when you're focusing on a balance while you juggle and your brain is otherwise occupied, they'll slowly creep up to catch the objects higher and higher. While many jugglers are at peace with this, it's bad form that will hinder your ability to progress. Keep your hands low, toward the line of your navel. The lower your catches, the more time you have to make corrections.

How should I go about learning to juggle four clubs with a balance?

Most people learn this trick in four-club singles. That is the wrong approach, assuming you'd like to learn some four-club tricks with a balance or move along to five clubs with a balance. Repeat the same "throw and catch" drills, but throw a club with a double spin. This will absolutely cross the top of the balance in your picture plane and can be confusing (and scary!) at first. Learning to juggle 441 with a balance, with the 4s as doubles, is also an excellent drill for this trick. Of course, this is beyond the scope of this little book. We'll get to club juggling and spin control in another volume some other time.

Yeah, but how do I master juggling with a balance?

I tell my students that the standard for "mastery" of juggling with a balance is 200 catches of five balls with a club balance. (The truth is, though, that there's no such thing as mastering any of this. There's advancing, there's becoming more proficient, there's getting it performance-ready... but there's always a harder skill. Even the most talented juggler would have a hard time qualifying seven balls with a teaspoon balanced on their nose!)

My neck hurts. Why are you hurting me, Thom?

If you're just getting started with this skill, you're using muscles that you probably haven't used before. (And when you're doing the two-minute dowel drills at the start, you're certainly using those muscles more than you ever would have!)

You may also be tilting your head back too much. Try taking some of the backwards lean into the thoracic vertebrae (your shoulders and upper back) instead of just hinging at the back of your neck and its cervical vertebrae.

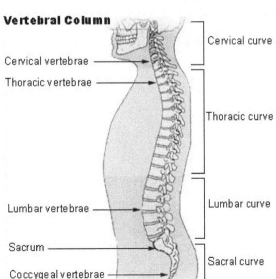

The vertebral column

Retrieved February 14th, 2020, from https://upload.wikimedia.org/wikipedia/commons/f/f8/Illu_vertebral_column.jpg
Public domain image.

Everything You Need to Know About Five-Ball Juggling

FIRST AND FOREMOST, the best props to use are the ones you've got. There's no silver-bullet juggling ball that will make your patterns better. When I first started working on five, I used misprinted Higgins Brothers beanbags. Then I moved on to 4" Dube stage balls. Then SportCo beanbags. Then russians. Then back to beanbags. And so on and so forth. None of those props made my patterns any cleaner—that's something that only practice can do for you.

That said, if you've got money burning in your pocket and you're set on buying a special set of props, I'd strongly suggest you use that as a reward. Can you qualify five consistently? Why not treat yourself to those balls after you've gotten 50 catches? Not there yet? How about buying that set after you get 20 cycles of all of your four-ball drills in a single practice session? It might sound cliche, but rewarding a milestone with a nicer set of props will really change the way you approach practicing.

If you're looking for prop recommendations, check out the appendix on different types of juggling balls!

Vocabulary

A **flash** of a pattern is n catches, where n is also equal to the number of objects thrown. So in the context of five-ball juggling, it means five balls thrown then caught. Depending on the context, some people refer to this as one side of a pattern.

The word "flash" can also mean making the throws higher for a designated number of throws, so you can do a pirouette underneath the pattern. Don't worry about this for now, though.

A **qualify** is twice as many catches as a flash, or "n*2." Speaking about five balls, this would mean 10 catches of a cascade pattern.

The **corner** of your pattern is where the ball peaks at the top of its arc—the point in space where you aim. When I talk about "placing" a throw, I mean a throw that intentionally peaks right in this spot. It's nice to think about delicately placing a ball there, rather than chucking in the general area.

The corner is an absolute point, over the vertical line of your shoulder. The difference between "corner" and "peak" is just that—we're talking about corners because it's an absolute. Every throw has its own peak, thanks to gravity. Not every throw reaches the corner of your pattern, due to our human fallibility—that's where practice and precision come in.

The **crossing point** is where the trajectories of throws in an odd-numbered pattern (3, 5, 7, etc.) intersect. A low crossing point tends to result in a wider pattern. A high crossing point tends to result in a slimmer pattern.

Siteswap notation is a system for writing down juggling patterns, measuring how long it takes an object to return to a hand after it has been thrown. (Some people use a shorthand and say that it's the throw height. Technically, that's wrong, but feel free to interchange height and time in this book. (Just know that it's wrong for now).

If you don't have a solid grasp on siteswap, now would be a good time to bone up on it. This book will get pretty siteswap heavy in a moment. If you're not familiar with it, head on over to Appendix A!

Starting Grips

When you start juggling with five balls, you hold three in one hand and two in the other. Starting a pattern with three in one hand can be a tricky thing when you first start. Let's clear up how to properly hold three balls in one hand.

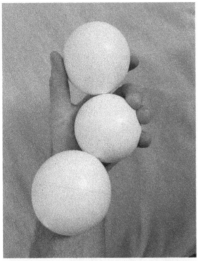

NO.
This is not the way to start. What are you doing?

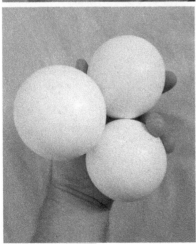

NO. This is also not the way to start.[20]

---

20 Fun fact: In Australia, some people call this the "NICA grip" because it's the way that an American juggling student insisted on starting it when he studied there. It was never advocated as the proper start by anyone at the school other than that one guy. Not naming names, but don't be like him.

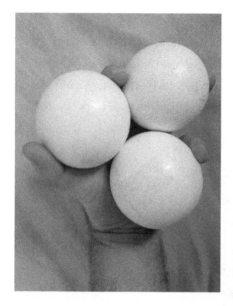

YES.

A triangle, with one ball held by the pinky and ring fingers, one held by the middle and index fingers, and one between the thumb and the palm.

The thumb ball is released first, then the index, then the pinky.

Easy!

Let's Get Serious

Enough with the little details. Let's get to work. You were probably wondering what I meant when I talked about four-ball drills earlier on.

Here's the thing (we're about to get a little cosmic here... step into my yurt and let's light some incense, all right?): The five-ball cascade is really a representation of your mastery of four balls. It's a representation of your overall juggling technique. It's not a one-off trick; it's a way of showing that you've put in some time and have a solid understanding of how juggling works.

A clean pattern happens because of a number of different factors. To run it smoothly, you need to have proficiency with accurate placement, an appropriate tempo, and a 5 height that's proportional to all of the other throw heights your body has learned (that's the siteswap 5—if you're not familiar with the topic, flip to Appendix A!) With a consistent three-ball cascade (siteswap 3) – or better yet, a consistent four-ball fountain (siteswap 4), you've got all of the tools you need to learn what a 5 looks like. That is, you'll know the exact height a 5 needs to be so that you don't have funny shifts in tempo or placement that cause you to correct.

A 5 that's too low effectively speeds up time—it'll make you rely on hand speed to continue with the pattern. (And that's a bad thing. If you want to progress, you need to grow technique that's founded on tall, beautiful throws. Relying on hand speed means being reactionary—you want to control the pattern, not have the pattern control you.)

"Okay," you say, "I'm going to leave this yurt unless you start giving me practical tips." Fair enough. Let's get to it.

A throw is like a vocabulary word. Learn to pronouce it well, then put it into a sentence. ("You had your warning, Thom. I'm leaving now!" "No, hold up! This will all come to a head in a second!") If our goal is to get a perfect five, let's work on some patterns that force you to attend to the 5 as it relates to throws you already know. Simple geometry. ("You're mixing metaphors. I'm leaving.")

Here are some of the best patterns to work on for the juggler who's about ready to flash five balls. (You'll probably recognize some of these from the three- and four-ball siteswap sections!)

5551

55514

534

7441

71 [21]

51

531

53

---

[21] If you choose to use 71 or 51 as training tools, use them to get a better understanding of height. The hand-scoop path of a shower pattern can be different than the motion used for a cascade.

You'll notice that I left out a few "standard" training patterns that other juggling books talk about—notably the snake (siteswap 50505), the three-ball flash (siteswap 55500), and 522.

...That's because those patterns all have 0s and 2s in them. If we're working on these patterns as a way to measure a 5 against other throws you already know, the method totally falls apart. How long does it take you to not throw a ball (Siteswap: 0) or to hold a ball in your hand (siteswap 2)? That's a hard question to answer, isn't it? (Maybe a Buddhist monk would know the answer. Want to climb a mountain with me later?)

Of the patterns I recommend, 5551 and 55514 are king. 5551—especially training it into and out of a four ball fountain (that is, 4444... 5551 4444...)[22] forces you to notice the relationship between the 5 and the 4 immediately next to one another. If you're throwing the 5s too high or too low, your tempo will be off when you re-enter the fountain. Drill this until it's starting to feel more comfortable (on both sides!), then start working on repeating the pattern (so—4444... 55515551 4444...) and then start working on getting the pattern to switch sides with a single 4 (that's 55514—so, 4444... 555145551 4444...) Rinse; repeat; level up.

I suggest the three-ball shower in both directions (siteswap 51) as a way to focus on the way your hand throws the 5. Are you doing a proper hand scoop, or are you catapaulting the ball? In order for this exercise to work, make sure you're actually completing the scoop, as you would when juggling five balls. Drill this, learn to switch sides (siteswap 51252) and see how it goes.

531 with the 1 behind the back is a way to really be honest about getting your throw heights solid. There's no way to cheat this one with handspeed, as your arms will be momentarily behind your back. It'll only work if the throws are nice and tall.

---

22 A quick note about ellipses: When we want to indicate an arbitrary number of throws or cycles of a pattern, we put an elipsis after the numbers. In this case, it does not matter how many 4-beat throws you make—the important thing is that a number of throws happen on either side of the siteswap we're training.

7441 is a great way to cross train a bit—if a 5 is a certain height, what's a 7? Really, just a super-tall 5, right? If you're working on these drills, you likely have a solid 441 with three. It can be helpful for some learners to learn what their natural 5 is by approaching it from the other direction—learn what a 5 *isn't*, as well.

These five-ball drills aren't in any particular order—some will be more challenging than others. Focus on one for a while, then start working on another. Working on a variety of these patterns at the same time will help keep you sane—and will make you a more proficient juggler, to boot. Not a bad deal at all.[23]

Preparing for your first Five Ball Flash

When you decide it's time to go for your first five-ball flash, here's your mantra: Place three, chuck two. You've got a lot of stuff to get out of your hands, so it's tempting to rush it. To counter this, think about placing the first three balls slowly into the corners of the pattern, then rush the last two (but *only* if you feel like you *need* to rush!). We're getting into the habit of a tall, slow pattern—accuracy and height over hand speed! Remember, if you have a solid 5551, you've already got a solid 555. A five-ball flash is just five 5s in a row, and you're already nailing the first three! Remember your tempo from the four-ball drills, place those first three 5s into their spot in the air, and if you've got to rush, only rush the last two. As always, height is your friend.

If you're already getting 10-20 catches with some regularity, here are some of my favorite drills:

---

23 These drills all have parallels with Richard Kennison's methodology when coaching juggling. He's a recipient of the International Jugglers' Association "Excellence in Education" award and knows what he's talking about!

• Clean five-ball flashes starting on each side (yep, you've got to learn to release three from your left hand, too! If you don't, how will you ever learn a six fountain?)

• Isolation training.[24] When I was teaching a past student how to juggle, she'd call this "juggle island" (and, I'll add, she hated it, because this drill can get extremely frustrating). Work on your five flashes and longer runs while standing on a chair. (Work on the four-ball drills this way, too!) Isolating your body in space will make you realize how much you're relying on corrections rather than perfect throws. It's sobering, but don't beat yourself up about it if you find it frustrating!

• If you're still in the 10-20 catch club, don't forget to work on your four-ball drills. When you practice those drills, you're also practicing five.

Can I skip from three to five without all of this four nonsense?

NO.

Onward and Upward

If you're already in the 50-catch club, it's time to start drilling the harder stuff.

Five-ball tennis is a personal favorite. That is, one ball thrown back and forth over the pattern as a reverse cascade throw. This is one of the drills that Richard Kennison, the juggling coach and IJA Educational Excellence award winner I mentioned earlier, preaches in his workshops. This drill forces you to attend to the reverse 5, leaving your lizard brain

---

24 Though you might recognize this as a traning tool advocated by Jason Garfield of the World Juggling Federation, the idea of isolating body movement has been around for a long time—it's been common practice at circus schools in Russia and the Ukraine for decades! Your humble author assumes no responsibility if you fall off a chair and hurt yourself.

(or muscle memory, or whatever you want to call it) to make the 5s that happen underneath it. This is a great drill to see how consistent your 5s really are. In the educational world, they'd describe this as a way to see if your explicit knowledge has gelled into implicit knowledge, to see if you've gotten to a level where your body does the action (here, the 5s under the reverse throw) without direct, conscious input.

Endurance. Your goal is a five-minute long run (that's roughly 1,250 catches). To build up to this level, you're going to have to build a little body muscle and a little brain muscle. Set a timer to five minutes and start running your five cascade. If you drop, pick up and keep going. Focus on clean throws that are placed where they should be. If you're feeling particularly motivated, do this drill at the start and end of every practice session.

Once you finally get a run of 2+ minutes, start working on this in isolation, with a balance, with a head bounce, or with anything else you can think of to add difficulty. When I started training endurance more diligently, I brought my personal best from 2 minutes to 20 minutes in about a month and a half. ("Will you juggle five balls for me for 20 minutes at the next festival I go to, Thom?" "Absolutely not. I was young and foolish back then. Much easier to tell you to do it instead.")

Notes and Caveats

Of course, these tips aren't the only way to train. Give them all a shot, and see what works for you! If you find the three snake (that's 50505) to work well, absolutely pursue it. The key to progress is pushing yourself and putting the hours in. Everyone's internal syllabus is different. (...But I will mention that I coached someone from zero juggling experience at all to 50 catches of five within six weeks using this method. She was super motivated, though, and the idea of proportional throws really jived with her learning style. Your mileage may vary.)

The Pyramid

One training method I didn't mention is the pyramid technique. I've never found it to work for me, but Warren Hammond, my former roommate and IJA Educational Excellence award winner, swears by it. No one method will work for everyone—the pyramid technique might be the key for you if some of the other drills we talked about didn't jibe.

Essentially, the pyramid technique is a sneaky way to get you warmed up with clean starts and finishes, slowly increasing the number of throws in each run. Here's an example of a pyramid-style training session:

Five ball flash: 20x clean.[25]
Seven catches: 15x clean.
Five ball qualify: 10x clean.
Twenty catches: 5x clean.
Fifty catches: 3x clean.

By the end of this particular example, you will have done 55 clean starts and finishes in a training session. If you're motivated by having a real, concrete way to track your progress, this might be a method you'd have success with. That said, my favorite training structure—"The Twenties"—is outlined in the next chapter.

Another tip that you might find helpful is learning to balance—check out the chapter on balance to get started with that. Balancing a dowel/club/shovel/whatever you've got around the house will train your body to understand its center line. That is, coincidentally, the same line where the balls cross in front of your body. Training this isn't exactly toss juggling, but your arms will need a break sometime (especially after you've done your endurance drills, right?). This is an extremely good skill that will serve you well as you progress with your juggling in the

---

25 Expert mode: alternating starting hands between each attempt.

future. You can find all of that information in the chapter "Learning to Balance" on page 67.

Training Method: The Twenties

"THE TWENTIES" are a kind of siteswap-based endurance training.

The gist is this: You pick a siteswap and run it for 20 cycles without stopping or returning to the base fountain or cascade. If you drop in the middle of the run, you have to start over again. Rinse and repeat until you succeed, then move on to the next siteswap.

Does that sound brutal? Yeah, it kind of is. It's monotonous and a bit mind-numbing... but it's a good way to stay honest about your training, and it helps you bulk up your juggley muscles.

But... why do you recommend this?

This series of drills helps you build up endurance and precision.

The tricky thing about siteswaps is that they're all about proportions. If everything is in perfect proportion, you'll be able to perform the base pattern (a four fountain or five cascade, for example), enter the siteswap, and return to the base pattern without any change in the rhythm (or "metronome") of your juggling. Human brains have their limitations, though, and it can be hard to tell by executing just one cycle if the siteswap was actually proportionate or not. It's possible that there was a slight anomaly that was too small to notice.

...So how can we start to notice these issues?

The Twenties are a way to magnify disproportionate throw heights and iron them out. It's almost like separation chromatography—taking a given pattern and examining where the impurities are—isolating them by allowing the errors to compound.

By repeating the pattern 20 times, the errors will compound, becoming much more pronounced (likely getting to a point where you drop!). If your 744 is plagued with high 7s and low 4s, the timing will deteriorate as you run the pattern—the pattern will get syncopated. The 7s and 4s may start landing at the same time, you may have to make big changes to the timing of your throws, or it might all just collapse all together.

The important thing about this drill is that you remain mindful of the rhythm of the base pattern before you enter the siteswap. After you complete the 20 cycles and return to the base pattern, is it syncopated or otherwise "off"? In a perfect world, the initial base pattern, the 20 cycles of the siteswap, and the base pattern you return to will all be on the same rhythm—all juggled to the same metronome.

An Important Reminder

The natural height and tempo of a base pattern varies from person to person. If you pick two five-ball jugglers out of a crowd and get them to execute a five-ball cascade side by side, their "native" height of the five-ball pattern will likely be different. Siteswap is all about proportions, and these drills are about learning the relationships of differing throw heights.

By working the pattern with endurance training, you'll be able to identify the issues and correct them as you practice. Or you'll just get frustrated, give up, and start a lucrative career in investment banking. Really, either outcome is a positive life improvement. (See? The Twenties are a great tool!)

Here are a few patterns that I suggest training with this method. They're listed in no particular order—try a few and see how it goes!

For 3	For 5	For 6
531	744	777771
441	663	9555
423	645	75
51	753	
	91	

For 4		
	66	771	3	
	97531	
7531	88441	
75314	75751	
7441	95551	
74414	8448641	
633	8642	
5551	(6x,4)*	
55514	(6,4x)*	
642		
71		
5	561	3		
534		

Okay, so how is this any different than normal endurance training?

The Twenties are good because they're a simple, measurable goal. If you're working on learning a seven-ball cascade, getting long, clean runs of patterns with five and six that incorporate 7 height throws will help you in that endeavor. In your daily training, you might noodle with a few different tricks, then move on. The fact that this drill forces you to achieve a given number of cycles before moving on makes you more honest about your training.

If you're rehearsing a routine for the stage, the Twenties are a great way to make sure that your material is rock solid. Many people practice routines just by running through their act and giving the most time and attention to their finale trick. Some of these performers drop in the "easy" parts of their routine on stage and wonder why. By addressing each and every trick in a routine with this drill, you get a much more realistic view of how clean you'll be on stage.

So, yes. This is "just" an endurance technique—but it's a framework that I've had a lot of success with. (It's also pretty similar to how I trained my act for Cirque du Soleil!) I hope you find it useful!

A Very Important Note

I'm absolutely not saying that this is the single greatest juggling drill of all time.

In fact, these days, I use this as a "filler" training method when I'm not feeling inspired or motivated. Do the drills, let the results be the results, and move on with your day. It combines siteswap training with endurance, so it's a good way to have a varied practice without thinking too hard and ensure you won't be slipping backward by taking a day off.

10 Ways to Make a Trick with Jay Gilligan

The game of making a trick easily starts with an instigation—some concept which can be applied without much initial effort, as a way to jump-start the process. Jugglers often relish making problems on purpose, and it's in the solving of these problems which leads to a new discovery. Each of the following starting points can be seen as a loose framework that gives a direction and suggestion that needs to be filled in with any number of details to produce a result. This type of construction solves the "blank-paper" syndrome of having so many possibilities that it's too overwhelming to even get started. And yet, these little conceptual approaches also allow a wide range of freedom to complete the process in many different ways, so the work will rarely get stuck once it gets going. While the strictness of applying each idea at the beginning might seem to be diametrically opposed to the looseness of figuring out the final outcome, this method means there will never be any hesitation or doubt about what the task is to accomplish—and yet surprises that occur along the way can be incorporated and utilized.

An added benefit of using conceptual suggestions is that they remove judgments of "good" and "bad" in relation to the material produced at first. The only exercise is to follow the chosen command and see where it leads. This is very closely related to the "Oblique Strategies" by Brian Eno and Peter Schmidt, a card-based method for promoting creativity, first published in 1975. Each card in the deck offers a challenging constraint intended to help artists break creative blocks by encouraging lateral thinking. A suggestion when working is to get all of the early (and most obvious) ideas out of the way first—and not as a mental exercise, but actually manifest them physically. Set a goal to make 10 variations of whatever concept is being employed. This permits enough permutations that results get produced immediately to fill out the list, and as 10 tries are added up, the ideas get progressively harder to find. It is in these later attempts that truly novel approaches often emerge. One thing to never forget with any of these methods—there is no one right answer! These ideas are theoretical, sometimes metaphorical, and rarely formally codified. They are simply inspirations and provocations to be taken seriously only as far as they keep the creative process moving forward.

1. Two Plus One

Since most basic juggling starts with three objects in a default pattern, this movement can already stop any critical thought process with the distraction of having to maintain what is happening before anything new takes place. Traditionally, jugglers have a habit of starting a pattern to enter into the creative process, perhaps trying to see what organically pops out—either as a "happy mistake" or a more intentional improvisation. Creating juggling certainly is a balance between considering a scenario and trying to already imagine what could happen, coupled with actual physical attempts to gain real-world feedback. Removing one of the objects from a three-object pattern and starting with the remaining two reduces the complexity and gives room for more a complex examination of potential moves. This lowers the technical barrier, and there is more time to think of what will come next. Compose a small sequence or even a single figure with two objects. Once you clearly and unambiguously establish something, add the third object back in. This process can be done in several ways, but the most important quality is to preserve the two-object trick as perfectly as possible. Obviously, changes will have to be made to incorporate the extra object, but the more intact the original pattern can be, the more effective this game is to play. One recommendation of how to add in the third object is to actually get rid of it as fast as possible—usually by doing a very high throw and then executing the two-object figure underneath before the first object comes down. This may not be the most eloquent approach, but sometimes it yields a great trick immediately! An extension of this trick creation concept can be to start with only one object instead of two, and then add in the next objects progressively, all the while keeping the first one-object pattern intact.

2. Prop Swap

One goal of modern juggling has been to make prop-specific technique—that is, tricks that can only be done with that discrete shape. Countless things can be thrown and caught, so a simple throw is not a good object-specific technique. But doing a scissor catch with clubs is something that is not traditionally translated to ball or ring juggling for example. A scissor catch, in its most basic form, relies upon the unique physical qualities of the club shape, catching a single club's handle between the bulbs of two other clubs held together in a hand. However, re-examining, and re-defining the properties of what qualifies as a scissor catch can be applied to anything, not just clubs. Instead of saying that two clubs are held by their handles side by side and are used to pinch the third club upside down by its handle, using its knob to stop it from falling vertically, one approach could be to look at the trick on a higher conceptual level and simply say two objects are trapping the third object. Then it becomes possible to find scissor catches with balls, rings, diabolos, or any other combination of three objects (foot, hand, wall, floor, etc.). Additionally, you can focus on any other detail of the scissor catch to creat parameters to explore with different props. Even if sometimes it seems as if this approach is simply a word game, the closer examination of what really constitutes the essence of a trick is richly rewarding. At first, doing a "ring pulldown" with clubs may seem impossible, but perhaps a pulldown simply means all the props end up sitting on the neck and shoulders instead of literally encircling the head.

Clubs and balls could easily be placed or trapped in these positions... a five-club pulldown would be a great exercise to try and accomplish! One of the best merits of this conceptual approach is that the starting tricks to investigate already freely exist everywhere. Therefore, the beginning of this process will never be exhausted.

3. Multiplex

Making a new trick does not always mean learning entirely new techniques. Every trick that already exists can have infinite variations. A straightforward way to modify an existing trick is to add multiplex. This can be done in any number of ways, with the two main strategies being to either add in more objects at the points of manipulation, or to combine the objects existing in the original pattern for a condensed version of the trick. Multiplex traditionally is defined as throwing two objects from the same hand at the same time. A modern definition of multiplex is more broad and states that any moment in time where there is more than one thing happening simultaneously can qualify as a multiplex. This definition generally still focuses on multiple props performing concurrent actions, but body parts and environmental aspects can also come into play.

4. Shape

Most juggling technique today stems from intuitive and unconscious traditions. These traditions include memes and trends of what is "acceptable" and valid inside the juggling community. This results in a limited scope when searching for inspiration. At present, juggling tricks generally exist in relation to other juggling tricks or at the very least strong juggling concepts: cascade, shower, reverse cascade, columns, body throws, pirouettes, siteswaps, body rolling, anti-spin, etc. But there are a limitless number of concepts to apply to juggling that come from outside the genre. Perhaps the most useful concept is the idea of shape or form. Jugglers normally organize objects in the air by patterns that are known and understood to be possible. Taking an outside image, such as a circle (or line, square, triangle, etc.) and organizing the objects according to that shape will give impressive results. First arrange the objects by the outcome you desire, and then begin to invent supporting techniques you need to hold that shape. Shapes are a powerful way to create tricks, since juggling is already a graphical art form. The American juggler, Dan Bennett, became famous for stabilizing three balls in an equilateral triangle, which hovered in the air in front of his chest during the Three-Ball Open at the 1989 IJA Festival in Baltimore, Maryland. More recently, Murakami Tsubasa from Japan made the image of juggling three-balls in a vertical line extremely popular in the current juggling zeitgeist.

5. Addition/Subtraction

Another "outsider" idea to apply to a pre-existing trick is the concept of addition and subtraction. This is loosely related to multiplex but has a very different choreographic intent. The main method is to literally hold an extra object, usually in a hand if possible, and not use it except for one moment in the trick, where it is released and incorporated in the action. This is the moment of "addition," after which the extra object is taken out of the pattern, back to its holding position, to accomplish the "subtraction." Of course, addition or subtraction can be done independently, without the couplet of the other. A basic example could be to juggle a three-ball shower while holding a fourth ball in the higher throwing hand. In the right timing, the fourth ball is briefly added to the pattern for one throw and then collected back to its original holding spot. It is in the release and collection technique that new tricks can often be found. The release lends itself to more traditional multiplex ideas, while the collect is often more foreign, since it's a collect that allows for other juggling to still continue, an idea not usually explored. The extra objects to be added to a pattern do not only need to be held in the hands; other body parts or the environmental architecture can be utilized. As well, the extra objects do not need to be the same kind of object as used in the base pattern—an especially fun combination can be to add a silicone ball into a pattern using beanbags, allowing for a bounce at one moment in an otherwise airborne form.

6. Rewind

As juggling is a relatively new art form, borrowing ideas from other art forms and applying them to juggling is not a futile process as of yet. Concepts from art forms which also deal with physical space and time are particularly applicable, such as dance. Compared to juggling, dance has a very rich and deep history, which can be explored by translating its development into juggling methods. The compositional idea of "rewind" yields such surprising juggling results, often going against very ingrained, natural, and intuitive technical juggling habits. The process is very straightforward—take an existing trick, move, or sequence and imagine as if it were a film being rewound. Most of the content will be physically possible (though perhaps technically insane) to execute in this manner, except some of it will absolutely not work due to gravity only working in one direction. It is of course impossible to rewind a move which relies upon gravity to work, as objects cannot "fall up" on their own. Once again, it is precisely these moments that give rich opportunities to invent solutions that solve these problems.

7. Five into One

This idea comes from the late Luke Wilson and was a favorite game of his when teaching juggling. First, a sequence of five different tricks is created. The tricks can be as basic or complex as desired; however, the second step may suggest a level of simplicity which allows for an easy technical execution of the original sequence. It does not help the game to make the five tricks overly "clever," and it's wise to include as much clarity as possible. This is because the second step of the game is to combine all the tricks into as few throws as possible. Ideally, all five tricks would be completed with only one common throw, but to achieve this level of perfection is essentially impossible. A good metric to attain is doing all five tricks with three throws total, and even this can rarely happen. A concrete example of how this can work might be a sequence that includes a pirouette followed by a run of backcrosses. One way to combine these two tricks could be to throw a backcross and pirouette underneath it, thus completing both tricks at the same time. Be careful not to "think ahead" when composing the original sequence, trying to imagine how the tricks might be consolidated and picking tricks based upon a hypothetical solution. The main benefit of this game is the surprise it lends to the trick creation process.

8. Helping Hands

Rhythm is perhaps the most important element for juggling. Rhythm is fundamental to the success (or failure) of all juggling technique. Since it plays such an important role, playing with the rhythm of a juggling trick can have a major impact, so much so that it creates what is seemingly an entirely new trick. Many tricks are related through hidden rhythmical concepts that jugglers today are barely aware of. Two patterns that seem to have no connection and which look completely opposite may actually be cousins in the world of juggling rhythm. A good example of how to play rhythm in juggling is to look at how any asynchronous pattern can be made into a synchronous pattern. An accessible way to manifest this is to take the work of one hand inside a juggling pattern and do that same amount of work with both hands together. Using the three-ball cascade as an example, each hand traditionally throws one ball every other beat. Extend the height of the throws and speed up the rhythm to the point where both hands can throw each ball in the cascade pattern on every beat. Essentially, this pattern could also be seen as "three balls in one hand," but now both hands are playing the role of the single hand here—and not as a metaphor, but actually literally and physically—both hands touch each other to form one larger catching and throwing surface and help each other to collect and release each ball. This game of turning the work of one hand into two hands can be done with any pattern and with any technique. Body throws are very fun to try with this method. Alternatively, it is possible to turn the work of two hands into one hand at various moments, again by using rhythm. This process is much simpler for resulting asynchronous patterns, and the higher challenge of translating a resulting synchronous moment while using one hand may give a bigger payoff in the long run. A nice entry point for turning the work of two hands into using only one hand is the stopping and collecting of all three balls in a three-ball cascade, without changing the direction of any of the throws. All three balls will end up in the same hand, but that hand will have to chase after each throw from side to side to end up with them all together.

9. Pain Charts

Pain Charts are also vaguely related to chance compositional forms inside the world of dance. Draw an even grid of squares that are approximately 1" on each side. Make the grid as large as the writing surface will allow. Across the top of the grid, write a repeating siteswap—for example, if 441 is chosen, write 441441441441, filling in each square with one numeral only until all the squares are filled. Down the left side of the grid, write a different type of juggling technique in each square until each square is filled. A list might include but is not limited to: under the leg, behind the back, bounce, hit, crossed arms, pirouette, balance, roll, trap, etc. Grab a small handful of rice, and sprinkle it across the paper indeterminately. Count the number of rice grains in each square, and determine which square holds the highest number of grains in each vertical column for the entire grid. The idea is produce a randomization of X and Y coordinates across the grid by which to match each siteswap throw with a juggling technique. The top of each column will tell which siteswap throw must be done, and whichever row has the highest number of rice grains in that column will give the matching way that siteswap throw must be done. For example, the spilled rice might have randomly determined that first 4 will have to be a bounce (off the floor, arm, wall, leg, etc.), the second "4" must be a hit, and the 1 should be a roll. It is then a straightforward process to evaluate the technical challenges to attempt the first three throws of this pattern.

This system often produces arcane results that are extremely technically challenging, but it forces jugglers to get out of the habit of repeating the same siteswaps with the same techniques. This means that, using the previous example, most jugglers would repeat 441 by doing a bounce, hit, and a roll, and then again do a bounce, hit, and a roll for the next 441. However, the "Pain Charts" method produces a different type of technique for each discrete throw—the first 4 in the first round of 441 might be a bounce, but in the second round of 441 the first "4" might be a backcross. This produces a tough mental challenge to remember what type of throw comes next, a problem that siteswap normally simplifies. It is this extra mental layer of memory added to the physical challenge that makes this method sometimes very "painful."

10. Fusion

Fusion is another example of crafting juggling not around a technical juggling pattern concept but rather another external force. Fusion could seem arbitrary at first, but at its core this idea plays with the physicality of juggling, which is something that is rarely done. Most juggling is focused on moving the objects in different ways. To achieve these movements, 99% of all juggling is done in a very practical way. Posture and stance are always formed from a utilitarian point of view. The juggling pattern itself might be made to be extremely complicated, but the body manifesting that pattern will be as efficient as possible to allow for technical complexity. No one ever juggles seven clubs with one eye closed or does five-club backcrosses standing on one leg. These would both be very hard tricks to do, but only because juggling culture does not count the variation of closing one eye or standing on one leg as valid criteria for a trick. If closing one eye was accepted as something a juggler can explore to add complexity to a trick, then the technique of closing one eye would be spread, practiced, and eventually incorporated into the general technique pool that new jugglers learn. Closing one eye would then end up not being a novel or foreign idea and lots of jugglers could (more) easily do it. Fusion is motivated by these cultural observations and is the simple idea of choosing to join two body parts together and exploring that physical reality while juggling. A favorite fusion is to "join" an elbow and a knee. The process by which to do this is to simply hold the elbow to the knee and not let them separate. Physical joints can be created with tape, straps, or perhaps other clothing, but an imaginary bond is just as useful. Fusion allows juggling to explore body architecture and, most importantly, the concept of negative space. Any two or more body parts can be used in a fusion, including more than one juggler.

Juggling in Front of an Audience with Fritz Grobe

AS YOU LEARN MORE and more tricks with three balls—and learn to juggle four and five—one question always starts to come up: What do you do with these newfound skills? At some point, almost every juggler wants to share what they've learned with an audience.

So how do you go from having a few tricks to having a routine that you can perform on stage? We'll take a look here at a method for building a routine that is ultimately set to music. However, many of these same principles apply to every kind of juggling act.

As with creating a new trick, if all you have is a blank stage in front of you, it can be difficult to know where to start. Every routine I've ever created has started with a small idea—something simple that intrigued me. It could be a trick I think is cool, like juggling while lying down; a gag I think is funny, like trying to juggle and drink a glass of water at the same time; or an image I think is beautiful, like juggling under an open umbrella. I've never had a piece spring fully formed into being. It's always started with that one small idea and grown over time. So start with something small that interests *you*, and see what happens when you explore it further.

When you first start working on a routine that will be set to music, the surprising recommendation is: Don't start with the music. Instead, start with your simple idea: that trick, gag, or image that excites you. From there, you'll create the building blocks of your routine, and then the music will guide you later on, when you put those building blocks together.

From Words to Phrases to Sentences to Paragraphs...

As you explore your simple idea, think of your basic building blocks as **words**: a throw under the leg, a pirouette, a siteswap.... Think of each trick as a word. Start to combine them into **phrases**: sequences of words, like a quick start into a shower into a pirouette.... Ideally, you are combining some of your favorite words to make interesting phrases. Those phrases combine into **sentences**, those sentences will make **paragraphs**, and those paragraphs will come together to make an entire **piece**.

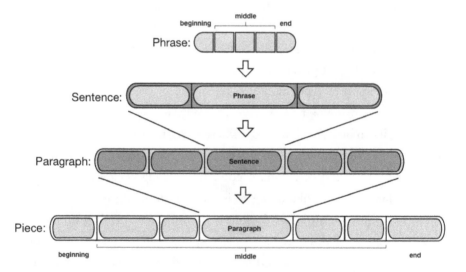

When making a new piece this way, you often don't know ahead of time what these words will "say," but that's okay. Take a trick you really like; see what happens when you combine it with another; and find transitions, movements, and ideas that build on those first words. Through that exploration, structures and themes often emerge naturally. These physical improvisations and discoveries are the lifeblood of a type of theater known as "devised theater."

Experiment with combining similar moves (like under the leg and behind the back) or contrasting moves (like rolling on the floor and juggling overhead).

Play with tempo: What's it like to do a trick faster or slower than usual? Look for opportunities to do two fast tricks in a row, or to switch between slow and fast.

Play with shapes: What's it like to do a trick bigger or smaller than usual? Higher or lower?

Try something. Then try something else. Start making a list of your favorite words and phrases—things you have tried that you like.

Structurally, each phrase will have its own beginning, middle, and end. If your phrase starts with a roll along the floor, where would you like it to end? High, low, slow, fast, big, small…? If your phrase will end with a pirouette, how could it begin? Try something. Then try something else. See what feels right.

From there, each paragraph will have a beginning, middle, and end. Does the "rolling along the floor" phrase start the paragraph? Does the "siteswap pirouette" phrase bring it to a satisfying conclusion?

Thematically, see which phrases have a distinct identity. For example, you might create:

- The "under the leg" phrase (a sequence of "words" that explore a progression of under the leg tricks).
- The "up to down" phrase (exploring moving from a trick up high to a trick down on the floor).
- The "circles" phrase (where each trick or word has a circular movement).
- The "rainy day" phrase (where each word is inspired by a feeling of rain falling).
- The "chaos" phrase (where you're moving as fast as you can from one crazy "word" to another).

You may find that you make phrases that are driven by structure, movement, imagery, or some combination thereof. There is no right way to do this, so explore all these methods and find what works for you.

Setting It to Music

Once you have built a collection of phrases, that's usually a good time to bring music into the process. The music will help you shape the piece. What music has the right tempo and feeling for your phrases? You may listen to dozens of pieces of music, testing each one out, before you find one that you think fits your phrases.

It's incredible how performing the exact same phrase of juggling tricks to different pieces of music can affect how you do that phrase and the way it feels. You may be able to do the same phrase slower and more lyrically, or faster and more percussively. Try showing a few phrases to a friend—each time to a different piece of music—and see how it changes the experience.

Once you have chosen a piece of music to work with, think about which juggling phrases fit with which parts of that music. When is the music small or big? When is it fast or slow? Which juggling phrases do you have that reflect that?

As you fit phrases to the music, how does each phrase need to be adjusted to work with the music? For example, you might find that the "under the leg" phrase matches a particular part of the music if you do four under the leg throws rather than two.

This is when creating a new piece moves back and forth between fitting existing phrases to the music and creating new transitions and new phrases inspired by the music.

Say the "up to down" phrase works perfectly for the beginning of the music, and that phrase ends with you sitting on the floor. Then the next part of the music fits the "circles" phrase, which starts with you standing and juggling overhead—but how do you get from sitting on the floor to standing and juggling overhead? Now that you are putting these phrases in sequence, you'll need to create a transition from one to the other.

You may also need to create whole new phrases. The "chaos" phrase may fit a particular spot in the music that's 15 seconds after the "circles" phrase—so now you need to create a new juggling phrase that will bridge that gap. All of this is part of the back-and-forth of combining juggling with music.

As the entire piece comes into shape, it will have its own beginning, middle, and end. Within that, there will be highs and lows, with rhythm and punctuation: a "comma" here, an "exclamation point" there…. Look for those opportunities for ups and downs, with variations of speed, movement, and feeling that will give your piece rich textures—a variety of images and impacts, with surprises that will help keep the audience engaged.

Choreographers will usually count out the beats of the entire piece of music, and each movement will be choreographed to specific beats. This is difficult to do with juggling and often isn't necessary. Particularly when you're starting out, rather than counting every beat, try choreographing to **anchors** in the music: Listen for key moments in the music, and anchor certain juggling words or phrases to those key moments. Then if you listen for those key moments, even if you drop, you can aim for the next anchor to keep the juggling phrases synchronized with the music.

If you find yourself getting ahead in the choreography—if you're early relative to an anchor—you can do a few extra throws to line up with that anchor and get back on track. And if you're late relative to an anchor, don't be afraid to skip a few words or even a whole phrase to keep the rest of the piece on track. Don't worry about making adjustments like these. You're the only person in the whole room who knows how the act is supposed to go!

Working with a Premise

Your piece may simply be driven by your specific choices, by the props, and by the music. That's great. But a premise may also emerge—a central idea that guides your choices. Your premise may be driven by technique ("I'm exploring body rolls"), movement qualities ("I'm contrasting circular and linear movements"), abstract imagery ("I want to evoke the feeling of rain in the forest"), or concrete imagery ("What if Beyoncé was a juggler?").

Famous jugglers have had many different motivations and styles. Francis Brunn combined flamenco dance with juggling. Michael Moschen focused on abstract shapes and integrating modern dance. Those premises then helped guide their choices of costume, props, music, and movements. If your premise is contrasting circular and linear movements, how could your costume reflect that? If your premise is evoking the feeling of rain in the forest, how could your props reflect that? What tricks and attitude would Beyoncé bring to juggling?

Ideally, every part of your piece should reflect that premise as much as possible.

For one of his pieces, my friend and Cirque du Soleil alumnus Steven Ragatz took inspiration from the work of painter René Magritte. That premise led him to wear a suit and a bowler hat; to manipulate large, solid-colored balls, briefcases, and umbrellas; and to use music and movement qualities that helped create a complete and consistent image. Every choice was driven by his central premise.

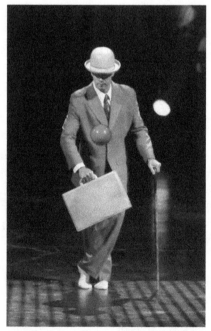

Again, you don't have to start with a strong premise like that to give you guidance. But look for those opportunities for your choices to be consistent with one another and to create a bigger picture.

As you build more and more pieces, your inspirations and methods will undoubtedly evolve.

Steven Ragatz in his signature suit and hat. Photograph by Jerome le Baut.

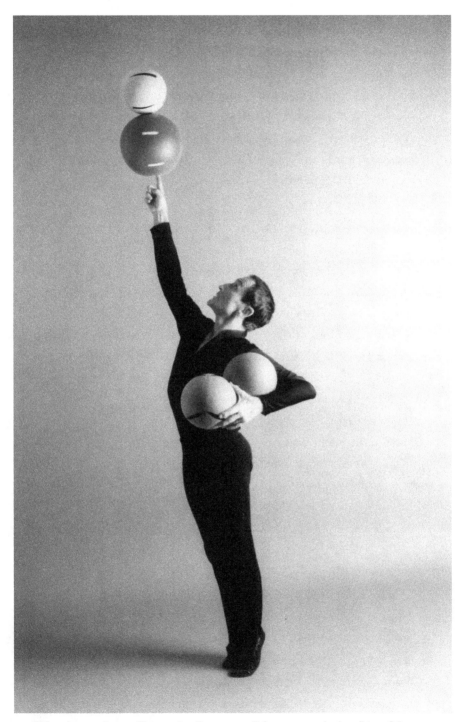

The legendary Francis Brunn. Photograph by Jim Moore.
www.vaudevisuals.com

You may find yourself starting with an overarching premise that guides your choices or with a specific piece of music that grabs you. You may find yourself counting every beat of the music so that it lines up perfectly with the juggling. You may be working on stage or on the street, silently or speaking. But in my own work, no matter what aspects of juggling I have found myself exploring, I have always returned in some way to building new words and phrases, listening for anchors in the music, and digging into strong premises.

A Quick Note about Costumes and Props

Thom uses the "Walmart Test" for costumes: If you wore the outfit and walked around Walmart, would people notice? If not, it's not a costume.

Steven Ragatz looks to create a unified, artistic look with his costumes and props. His suit, briefcase, and umbrella fit his René Magritte imagery. But when a different piece involved manipulating big boxes, he wore a set of coveralls and the boxes were made to look like shipping boxes—a completely different but equally consistent look.

Most of all, make sure your props will be visible. You want people to be able to see what you're doing! This means the colors of your props should contrast with both your background and your costume. Don't juggle white balls and wear a white costume!

A Conversation with the Audience

An easy trick can be interesting. A difficult trick can be boring. A great technical juggler can be dull to watch. And a less strong juggler can be an absolute joy. How does that happen?

For me, the fundamental metaphor for being in front of an audience that I find useful is that a performance is a conversation. Even if I'm not speaking at all, my goal is for the experience of being on stage with an audience to feel like a one-on-one conversation. We are connected and having a good time, together.

A conversation begins with two things: First, I have something to say; second, I am listening.

That means it all starts with something that I think is interesting. If I'm not genuinely interested in what I'm doing, how can I expect someone else to be interested? As Avner Eisenberg (Broadway's "Avner the Eccentric" and one of my teachers) says, "Don't try to be interesting; be interested." That's why I make sure every piece I do is driven by ideas that I personally think are exciting, from that trick I think is cool to that image I think is beautiful.

Variety performers sometimes have an attitude that says, "Look at what I can do that you can't." That's like a conversation with a know-it-all who doesn't really care about who he's talking to—he just wants to show you how smart he is.

But listening—making it a dialogue—means that you are paying attention to what others think and feel during your performance. Are they restless? Are they amazed? Are they uncomfortable, laughing, angry, crying…? Do their reactions match your objectives?

A good conversation has a nice, comfortable pace, comes to a natural end, and leaves everyone wanting more. If we get bored, the conversation moves on to something new. And before we feel exhausted with one another, the conversation comes to a satisfying conclusion, leaving us eager to see one another again.

A good conversation is relaxed. We are all breathing easily, without tension. It is difficult to bring that feeling onto the stage. The moment we step in front of people, we naturally tense up and hold in our breath. It takes practice and experience to keep breathing calmly and to make easy eye contact rather than looking at the floor or over the audience's heads. Relaxing, breathing, looking at each other—these things that we naturally do in conversation take time and practice to do on stage.

So do you have something you're eager to say? Are you listening and letting our reactions affect your responses and your timing, even in subtle ways? Are you prepared but ready to improvise? Rather than just going through the motions, are you genuinely here, now, in this moment with us?

You may go on stage and do your easiest trick and blow people away. Or you may do something insanely difficult and the audience is totally unimpressed. In the end, it is not so much about the tricks but about the feeling you give us in this conversation. Those tricks are your reason to be on stage. All that skill and preparation make you the person to watch. But then it becomes about how you make us feel. At the end of the conversation, do we feel like we've gotten to know each other?

Ultimately, this conversation is a chance to do just that: to get to know each other and to spend time together. To me, the best performers are ones who leave us feeling like we have become friends.

Practicing for Performance

Juggling in front of people is a lot harder than juggling in private, and catching that trick every single time is a lot harder than catching it on the 11th or 12th try for the video camera. Then throw in lights when you're inside, wind when you're outside, rain, sun, no opportunity to warm up, distractions…. Performance is great at making you drop.

Gus and Ursula Lauppe, my juggling mentors, thought a trick was only ready to try in front of an audience when they could do it in practice 9 out of 10 tries—and they were happiest when each skill they performed was 10 out of 10 in practice.

Ideally, what you present on stage is much less than what you can do in practice. Gus's typical solo warm-up was 200 catches with six rings, three times in a row. And he expected to be able to do that without dropping—and often without moving his feet or even making a major correction in the pattern. Then on stage, he would do only a short run of six rings and a flash of eight rings—a small fraction his skills off stage.

Now, the success of your performance may not depend on showing just how comfortable you are with six rings, the way Gus Lauppe did, but whether you are doing under the leg with three balls or flashing eight rings, the goal is to make sure that you are confident with what you are performing.

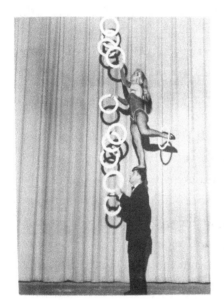 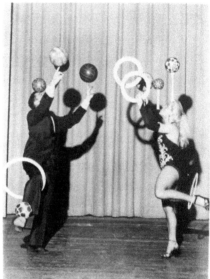

GUS & URSULA   CONTINENTAL JUGGLING ARTISTS

Gus and Ursula Lauppe perform.
From Fritz Grobe's personal collection.

The goal is to get your technique to the point where you will be surprised if you drop in performance—and you will still be comfortable in front of people if you do.

Three tactics for getting ready to perform a trick on stage are:

1) Try the trick 10 times in a row each time you practice. The goal is to reach the point where you are consistently catching it 9 or 10 times out of 10. If you're feeling particularly ambitious, consider making a spreadsheet to track your progress over time.

2) Practice something twice as difficult. If you want to do a pirouette, can you do two in fast succession? Do *that* 10 times each practice. If you want to do 10 catches of five balls in front of people, can you do 20 reliably in practice? That will give you more comfort and confidence when you want to do the easier trick on stage. If you follow Gus and Ursula Lauppe's example, you will be practicing some tricks that are 10 times as difficult as what you perform.

3) Practice the trick in sequence. If you want to be able to perform 12 catches with three-ball backcrosses into 12 catches of shoulder throws into a pirouette, practice each trick separately, then practice the entire sequence. To really get a sequence solid, practice each individual trick 10 times in a row, practice something twice as difficult as each individual trick, then practice the entire sequence. And yes, practice the entire sequence 10 times in a row, and for good measure, practice something twice as difficult as the entire sequence. Whew! All that to get one sequence ready to perform.

This can seem daunting, but the good news is that all you have to do is put in the work.

That's what I did to get my diabolo routine ready for the International Jugglers' Association championships in 1993. My practices included doing one "sun" with two diabolos 10 times in a row, then doing four suns ("Practice something ~~twice~~ *four times* as difficult") 10 times in a row, then doing my "sun phrase" ("Practice the trick in sequence") 10 times in a row, then doing my "double sun phrase" ("Practice something twice as difficult") 10 times in a row. All that to do just one sun phrase on stage.

Eventually, I was getting comfortable enough with every word and phrase in the piece that I could focus only on practicing the entire piece and working on any problem spots. But it took months of practicing to get there.

By the time the competition rolled around, I had practiced enough that I expected not to drop. That confidence was a big help, so when the big night came and I did have a drop, it didn't faze me and I was able to get right back into the routine.

Finally, **if you are having trouble with a trick, cut it.** That doesn't mean take it out of your piece forever. Keep practicing that tough trick, but only put it in your performance when it's ready. For the competition in 1993, everything in my piece was feeling solid except for three diabolos. So I cut it. Then I wasn't worried—"Uh-oh, here comes that shaky trick!"—and it made the whole piece better.

The goal is to be able to walk out and comfortably do your entire piece, start to finish, catching each trick in sequence on the first try, without worrying that you will drop.

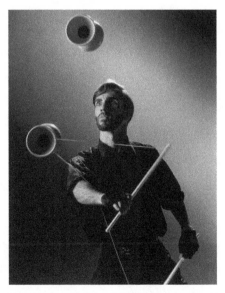

Fritz Grobe and his IJA-winning diabolos.
Photograph by Kent Phillips.

Dealing with Drops

Preparation is the best plan. Again, the goal is to practice to the point where you will be surprised if you drop any of the tricks you have chosen to perform. But no matter how much you practice, if you perform long enough, you will drop. You will drop on some difficult tricks. You will drop on some easy tricks. You will drop in new and surprising ways. I dropped once before I even started throwing. Drops happen.

When you do drop, you want that to be as relaxed as the rest of your performance.

Your technical practice should make sure those drops are as rare as possible, and your performing skills should make those drops as fun and inconsequential as possible.

The natural instinct when making a mistake in front of people is to freeze. You reflexively suck in a lungful of air and think, "Aah! What do I do next?!" It takes experience and a lot of practice to get past this instinct. Practicing what you do when you drop will help prepare you so you do indeed know what to do next, and experience will show you that you can survive all sorts of mistakes.

The key to handling drops well is in reacting calmly and comfortably. When you make a mistake, the audience will look to you to see if it's a problem or if everything is okay. If you're freaking out, the audience will, too. If you're calm and collected, the audience will follow your lead and go, "Oh, that's no big deal."

I've had people congratulate me for a flawless performance even when there were several drops. They forgot I dropped, simply because I didn't let those drops throw me. And when I've gotten a bit rattled on stage, I've had people say, "Boy, that looked rough!" even when nothing actually hit the floor.

Again, you're the only person in the whole room who knows how the act is supposed to go, so if you stay calm about any mistakes, so will the audience. As you perform more and more, you will accumulate ways of dealing with drops and, hopefully, become increasingly comfortable with this inevitable aspect of juggling in front of people.

Here are a few tips:

• First, don't panic. Just keep breathing.

Your continued breathing shows your comfort. If you suck in a lungful of air in panic, so will the audience.[26] Once, when I spectacularly dropped a prop off the edge of the stage, just by giving a big exhale, the audience was able to relax, empathize with my struggle with this difficult trick, laugh, and we all moved on just fine.

Part of "don't panic" is "don't rush." Our instinct when we make a mistake is to run around, pick everything up in a hurry, and get back to juggling as quickly as possible. It's a powerful instinct, but when you rehearse, it's possible to practice overcoming this instinct. Even when you're bounce juggling seven balls and all seven of them collide and bounce off in different directions, don't run around in a panic. Practice staying calm as you go around to collect them all. It will put your audience at ease and also keep you calm so that you don't rush from one mistake into another.

• Second, don't ignore it. Just deal with it.

The audience's focus will go toward the prop that is rolling along the floor. If you leave the prop where it fell and just move on to the next thing, the audience will still be thinking about that prop on the floor. Simply walk over calmly, pick it up, and continue. If you are a talking performer, a quick joke can acknowledge what happened, put people at

---

26 Bacrach, Fontbonne, Joufflineau, and Ulloa. "Audience entrainment during live contemporary dance performance: physiological and cognitive measures". *Frontiers in Human Neuroscience.* Vol 9. 2015. p179.

ease, and bring their focus back to you. But that joke may not even be necessary if you are calm and collected.

- **Rule of thumb: Only try a trick once or, maybe, twice.**

When you drop, either pick it up and move on to the next trick—no worries—or go back and give that trick one more try. Only on rare occasions should you try a trick more than twice in front of an audience, usually only when it's your last trick in a piece.

The danger of trying a trick three times is that if you miss it three times, it starts getting awkward. The audience starts to wonder how many times you're going to try it—and if you'll ever actually catch it. It's best to acknowledge, even silently, that the trick isn't happening right now and simply move on, making it no big deal.

When it comes to the last trick in your piece, it's harder to walk away without catching it. That's one reason you generally don't want to make your last trick your most difficult trick—make it one that you are extremely confident and comfortable with. Even then, it's a good idea to have a backup plan for when you miss your last trick. You can have an easier trick ready as an alternative ending in case you miss the more difficult one.

I have seen people break this rule of thumb, often with painful consequences, but once to great effect. The Gibadulin jugglers, a troupe of Russian club jugglers, finished their routine with six people tossing a grand total of 24

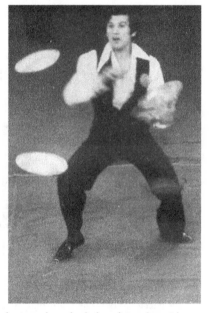

Damir Gibadulin catches plates hurled by his family. Adapted from http://www.ruscircus.ru/forum/uploads/post-0-1204066765.jpg

plates. They threw them like Frisbees all the way across the circus ring to one person who caught and collected them all into a tall, precarious stack. It's a big, beautiful trick that fills the space, with many plates in the air at any given time.

For this grand finale, on the 22nd plate, he missed, and the entire stack came crashing down. That first mistake may have been on purpose, to build tension. But then he missed on the next attempt. And the next. And the next. Altogether, that night in Radio City Music Hall, they tried the trick nine times—a recipe for disaster. Each time, the audience counted, "…18, 19, 20, noooo!" as the plates crashed down again.

Now, the Gibadulin jugglers knew they could get it. And they stayed calm. They kept breathing. It was a big risk, but it paid off. On the ninth try, "…21, 22, 23… 24!" The audience, which had been getting frustrated and worried for several minutes, rocketed to their feet with applause. The genuine, exhausted joy of the performers was explosive.

But trying until you get it is a dangerous game to play, and it will more often end with awkwardly giving up rather than spectacularly succeeding. While every rule can be broken, only trying a trick once or twice is usually best.

- **Even if you missed, make it a success.**

Sometimes catching 23 out of 24 plates is good enough.

Particularly when your five-ball pirouette was almost perfect but that last ball just slipped out of your hand, learn to notice when the audience thinks you succeeded, and let it be a success. Calmly pick that ball up off the ground, give it a little toss, and catch it firmly with an attitude that says, "Yes, I caught it!" Again, the audience is looking to you to know how they should react. If you can project an honest feeling of success, the audience will embrace that, and you can all move on to the next thing.

• **Finally, I'll say it again: Don't panic. Just keep breathing.**

This not only sends the right signals to the audience that everything is okay, it sends the right signals to your own body that everything is okay. If you rush, it's easy for one mistake to turn into another, and another... Take a moment; take a breath. Use that breath to refocus yourself. Let go of that mistake, be present in the moment, visualize what you're supposed to do next, keep breathing, and just do it.

Make Practicing, Writing, and Rehearsing Three Separate Activities

I've found it effective to separate out technical practice, writing new material, and rehearsing a piece. These are separate activities that should happen at separate times, but it can be easy for one to interrupt another and derail the task at hand. Be aware of that and give each of these tasks the focus it needs.

Practice is when you drill your technique and practice your tricks. Writing is when you explore new ideas, whether that's coming up with a new trick, a new joke, or an entirely new piece. And rehearsing is when you take what you've written and go through it as if you are in front of an audience. Each of these tasks benefits from dedicated time and attention.

In particular, don't stop a rehearsal to practice a trick that's giving you trouble. Don't interrupt rehearsing a piece to write a new bit. Yes, you want to make a note that the trick needs work or that you have a new idea. But finish the rehearsal first, then turn your attention to what's giving you trouble or where you can make an improvement.

The goal of a rehearsal is to practice what you will do on stage, in front of an audience. You won't stop in the middle of a performance to practice a trick, so don't do that in rehearsal. Rehearsal is when you see how you will deal with that drop. Rehearsal is when you make sure you know how you will handle a difficulty. Do you go back and try it one more time, or do you just move on?

Rehearsal is also when you make sure you're ready for the realistic circumstances you'll be in on stage. You won't necessarily have had the chance to warm up for 15 minutes right before. The lights may be bright and in your eyes. Your costume may cause an unexpected problem. Whenever possible, rehearse in spaces and circumstances similar to where you will be performing, so you can get used to that new costume, that lower ceiling, or those bright stage lights.

Next Steps

You can spend as much time (or more) working on your performance skills as on your juggling skills. Taking dance classes, acting classes, and improv classes can be a big help, even when you may not see immediately how those skills transfer to the performance of juggling. Just getting used to being on stage in many different ways—from open mic nights to improv shows, from clown workshops to dance recitals—will make you a stronger performer and can open up new ideas for presenting juggling to an audience.

Thom Wall, Steven Ragatz, and I—along with many other jugglers and variety performers—have studied at Celebration Barn Theater in South Paris, Maine. This school for physical theater offers many different workshops that can help you create new work and become a stronger performer.

Finally, the renowned mime and physical theater teacher Carlo Mazzone-Clementi created a list of four things that make for a great performance that are also part of the philosophy of performance at Celebration Barn:

- **Effort:** Be prepared and throw yourself into your performance.
- **Risk:** Let us feel that excitement, which is inherent to great juggling.

- **Momentum:** Whether your pace is fast or slow, give us a feeling of growing momentum.
- **Joy:** Ultimately, it's about spending time together and having this shared experience.

So, keep creating new pieces and performing as much as you can. There is no substitute for the experience of pursuing these four objectives in front of an audience over and over and over again.

ETHICS IN JUGGLING – DON'T BE A THIEF!

Most moves of every juggling routine are standard—that is, they are patterns that countless jugglers have used for decades, or even centuries. But the number of variations one can work with three, four, or five objects is, if not infinite, sufficiently vast for everyone to find a signature pattern. The signature pattern is the juggler's own invention, the one move he or she has discovered, and wrought to perfection. It is the one part of the routine where even the novice of one year might have something to offer to the veteran of twenty. Bobby May's drum trick, Fields' cigar boxes, Dimitri Karamazov's "I can juggle anything" challenge—these are all new contributions to the tradition which bear the stamp of the innovator's personality.

- Arthur Chandler, "On the Symbolism of Juggling: The Moral and Aesthetic Implications of the Mastery of Falling Objects" (Chandler, 1991)

THERE'S A LOT OF WONDERFUL juggling at your fingertips—right there on YouTube, Juggling.TV, and a ton of other sources. You might be tempted to learn someone else's material—and that's okay—provided you understand how to do it ethically. There are certain tricks, moves, and combinations that are considered "stock"—juggling three torches on a tall unicycle, for example (though some critics will say that a "stock" trick is just one that's been stolen by a lot of people). However, many performers have trained for years to create their signature style, unique tricks, and spectacular routines. Learning and performing someone else's routines is not okay.

Juggling comedian Scotty Meltzer offers a simple test for whether something is plagiarized or not—could you reasonably perform the same stunt or use the same line in a show with your "inspiration" and the audience wouldn't see the similarity?

In Scotty's article "Thou Shalt Not Steal," written for the International Jugglers' Association's online magazine, he proposes a thoughtful method for ethically "switching" material that you'd otherwise want to steal. Though he proposes the exercise for verbal comedy, it can also be used to recreate juggling tricks or routines in a unique way. Scotty's steps are as follows:

1.   Write down a joke you want to steal.

2.   Write down what makes that joke funny.

3.   Write examples that express your answer from step 2.

4.   Choose a few you think are funny and turn them into complete, performable jokes.

5.   Verify that you've switched that joke all the way to the bone.

6.   Off the page and onto the stage.

(Meltzer, 2012)

For our purposes, we'll use these modified steps:

1.   Select a sequence or stunt you want to steal.

2.   Write down what makes that sequence or stunt interesting.

3.   Write examples that express your answer from step 2.

4.   Choose a few you think are particularly interesting and turn them into complete, performable sequences or stunts.

5.   Verify you've switched the sequence all the way to the bone.

6.   Off the page and onto the stage (after some rehearsal, of course!).

Let's say you're inspired by some famous performing juggler's sequence where he starts by throwing three balls up in the air and doing a pirouette underneath them. Then he goes into a sequence where he throws them behind his back while gyrating his hips and moving his tongue in and out like a lizard. He finishes by throwing one high, placing two on the ground, then catching the last one on his neck and lying down flat on the stage. Here, we've done the first step—putting the pen to the page and describing our source material.

Step 2: What makes this sequence interesting? You certainly can't steal the sequence as a whole and claim it's your own—this is a fellow juggler's signature sequence, after all! The components certainly must be a surprising start and finish, interesting body movements, and throws coming from around the body.

Step 3: Let's find a list of tricks and sequences that are interesting for the same reasons as our source material. Instead of throwing all three up in the air from one hand and doing the pirouette, could you have them drop from the ceiling? Perhaps you could throw three up in the air from one hand and claw two from the air as they're going up. How about a more complicated start where all three are thrown in the air so they form a column, and you find a way to execute a pirouette as you catch each ball?

In terms of body movement, instead of a "juggler-as-gyrating-lizard," how might it look if the juggler were sailing on a boat? What about a drunk juggler? A shy juggler? A robot juggler? A prima ballerina juggler?

Instead of throwing the balls behind the back like our source, how about another part of the body? Under the leg or around the neck? There are infinite possibilities here.

Now let's move on to step four and test them out in rehearsal. What feels like it works?

Step 5: Record yourself doing your new sequence. Watch it. Then watch the source video. Could these two acts reasonably fit into the same variety show? If not, identify the parts that seem too similar and find other ways to follow the same reason why the thing is interesting, making it different from the original material. Rinse, repeat.

Step 6: Take your new routine to a local open mic, variety show, or other stage and see if it works.

One Big Important Note

...many circus schools have students "copy the masters" as an exercise. Since these exercises are closed to the public and the students don't try to pass this work off as their own, it's totally acceptible. Copying an existing work as a way to experience someone else's relationship to the choreography can be a valuable experience—it's all about the context.

APPENDICES

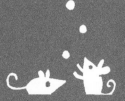

APPENDIX A: SITESWAP: THE LANGUAGE OF JUGGLING

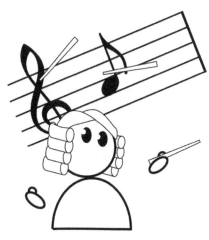

SITESWAP NOTATION IS A WAY that jugglers write patterns down. It was invented (or discovered—depending on who you're talking to, that could be the start of a big, pedantic argument!) in 1981 by a man named Paul Klimek. Originally known as "Quantum Juggling," siteswap got its name from juggler and mathematician Bruce "Boppo" Tiemann, one of several jugglers who were on the same track as Klimek but didn't quite crack the nut, so to speak (Åberg, 2018). (We're not going to get into a discussion about emergent intelligence, but it's amazing that there was more than one mathematician-cum-juggler figuring this out at the same time. Suffice it to say that siteswap is an important tool that has shaped the face of modern juggling!)

Siteswap changed the way jugglers describe juggling patterns to one another—the conversation went from "throw a ball kinda high on one side to the same hand, then one with the other hand at the same height to the same hand, then pass one underneath those two while they're in the air from one hand to the other, then throw that ball again like a normal juggling throw and keep doing a cascade after that" to "do 441333." Useful, right?

When written, siteswaps look like a string of incoherent numbers to the untrained eye. 441, 97531, (6x,4)*… complicated stuff at first glance. So let's look a little longer and break it down.

In music, written notes indicate how long a particular sound is played. You have full notes, quarter notes, eighths, and so on. In juggling, the number represents how long it takes for an object to return to a hand (or, perhaps more eloquently, the amount of time it takes for a ball to be re-thrown). Lots of jugglers will use a shorthand, saying that the number means how long an object is in the air—that is, the height of the throw. Though that's technically incorrect, we'll be using the idea of number value and height interchangeably in this chapter.

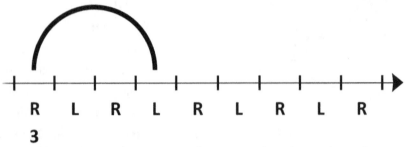

R   L   R   L   R   L   R   L   R

3

A three-beat throw goes from one hand to the other.

When you juggle a three-ball cascade, all of the throws are siteswap 3. That means that every thrown ball returns to a hand after three beats. A beat is an arbitrary measure of time—every juggler has their own internal metronome. Though it's usually considered best to have tall, slow patterns, if you get two jugglers to juggle three balls side by side, their patterns will almost invariably have slightly different tempos. My 3 might be different than your 3.

…Part of this is due to throw height, but the other part is due to something called dwell time—the refractory period where the ball is resting in your hand. If you're juggling three balls in a cascade with a long dwell time or if you're juggling three balls in a cascade with a short dwell time, the throws are all still the same. Imagine a metronome that marks time with a short click and a metronome that marks time with a longer tone—it's kind of like that. (If you're interested in learning more about this, and the more-complicated-than-we-need-to-get-here aspects of juggling math, check out Shannon's Theorem).[1]

> All that said, the big takeaway for our purposes is that *you've got an internal metronome that clicks out beats.*

The three-ball cascade is a relatively low pattern where everything crosses. As you probably know, the four-ball fountain is a different pattern!

Why do we juggle odd numbers in a cascade and even numbers in a fountain? Well, let's dive in!

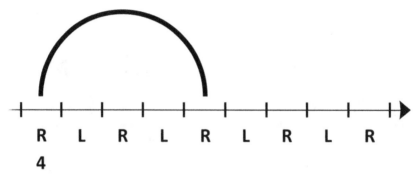

A four-beat throw returns to the hand that threw it.

When you juggle a four-ball fountain, all of the throws are siteswap 4. That means that every ball returns to a hand after four beats.

When you juggle a five-ball cascade… (and I think you know where I'm going with this now…) all of the throws are siteswap 5. A six-ball fountain? They're all 6s. A seven-ball cascade? They're all 7s. And so on and so forth.

Looking at the diagram on the following page, you might notice something. All of the odd-numbered throws cross the body—they're thrown and caught by different hands. All of the even-numbered throws stay on the same side and are thrown and caught by the same hand. Weird, right? Well, there's a reason for it!

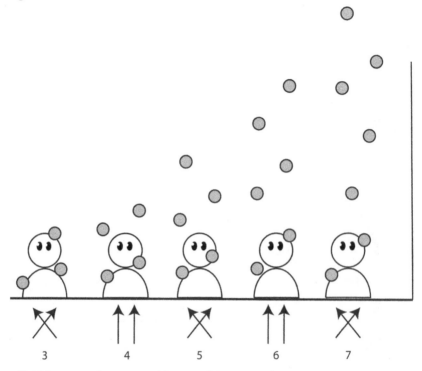

Different throws, all marching to the same metronome.

There are a few rules in siteswap, and the most important are that we must notate everything that happens on every beat (even if there's nothing for that hand to do in that time!) and that your hands alternate beats. This means that when you look at a string of numbers, they're alternating hands:

Right, left, right, left, right, left...

...Or, left, right, left, right, left, right... if you're left-handed. (Ha!)

So, if you're throwing an object for an odd length of time—throwing a 3 or a 5 or a 7 – the object can't be caught by the same hand that threw it.

If you're throwing an object for an even length of time—throwing a 4 or a 6 or an 8—the object must return to the same hand that threw it.

The bigger the number, the longer the object takes to return to a hand. In toss juggling, people often use that shorthand I mentioned earlier, just saying that a bigger number means a higher throw. (If you'd like to learn how to apply this idea, check out the chapter called "Everything Can Be a Hand: Applying Siteswap" on page 89!)

If this is all confusing, don't worry! It took juggling scientists the better part of four thousand years to arrive at this system—they figured this out so we didn't have to. (Let's hear it for someone else doing the work!)

The big takeaway here is this simple rule:

Odd throws switch sides. Even throws stay on the same side.

But Thom... what about the siteswap 2? What about 1? And 0?

Excellent questions!

A 2 is a throw that returns to the same hand after two beats. Knowing

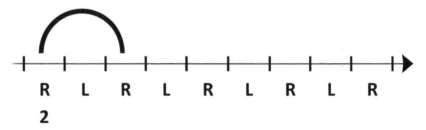

A 2 returns to the same hand—before that hand can do anything else. It can be held or thrown.

that we're always alternating hands, if a 2 starts in the right hand, it'll return to the right hand before that hand can do anything else. Thus, a 2 is an object that stays in the same hand—it's a handhold. (At least, that's what we're going to say for now. You can actually do a lot with a 2! But let's not get ahead of ourselves.)

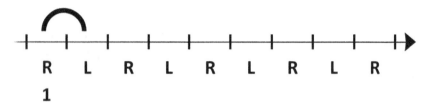

A 1 goes from one hand directly to the other.

A 1 is a throw that is caught exactly one beat after it's thrown—it's only in the air for a very small period of time. It's odd, so it crosses. What's the fastest way to get a ball from one hand to the other? Simply handing it across—transferring the object as though you were clapping your hands together.

A 0 is an object that returns to the same hand 0 beats later. Sounds impossible, right? That's because it is! A 0 is the absence of an object—it's a placeholder that means that nothing happens in that hand in that beat, since there is no object present.

Let's Mix Things Up

So far, we've just talked about the base patterns: 333 with three balls, 444 with four, and so on. When you go to a symphony, things get interesting when there's more than one note that's being played. In the same way, juggling gets a lot more interesting when you use more than just one throw.

The very first pattern that was invented (or discovered!) using siteswap notation was a three-ball pattern called 441. Let's break that down.

Remember the example at the beginning of this chapter, where we talked about jugglers ages ago using descriptions like "throw a ball kinda high on one side to the same hand, then one with the other hand at the same height to the same hand, then pass one underneath those two while they're in the air from one hand to the other"? That's this pattern! That's 441!

4, right hand: Throw this ball kinda high on one side to the same hand

R   L   R   L   R   L   R   L   R

4   4   1

441 (Or: up, up, hand-across)

4, left hand: Then do the same thing with the other hand, straight up and down

1, right hand: Then pass one underneath those two while they're in the air, from one hand to the other

(But wait… what about that 1 again? This is still confusing!)

Well, what does siteswap mean, again? The numbers represent the length of time that an object takes to return to a hand after it's been thrown. A 1 crosses from hand to hand (it's an odd-numbered throw), returning to a hand after one beat. Since we always alternate left and right hands, there's nothing that the receiving hand could do in that time. So, a 1 is literally passed from one hand to the other.

441 is an incredible pattern, as it requires that you learn a 4 using the same beats—that is, the same metronome—as your three-object cascade. Assuming that the duration of your beat is always the same (and you've got great technique, after all—let's make that assumption!), a 4 needs to land exactly one beat later than a 3 would. To execute this pattern from a three-object cascade and back with a perfect rhythm (that is, without any kind of stutter or shift in the beat), the 4 needs to be perfect.

Yes, you could achieve some form of juggling success by shifting your metronome around to accommodate imperfect throws… but in doing so, you're learning bad habits. If you want to progress to more complicated patterns or higher numbers, you need to cultivate perfect, proportional throws.

For this reason, 441 is an excellent training pattern for a four-object fountain. The fountain—the base pattern for four objects—is just a four-beat throw executed again and again. 441 teaches you how to make a four-beat throw perfectly, measuring it against your 3—a throw you already have ingrained in your body.

An Important Note About Notation

When you say 441 to a juggler, you're literally just saying a sequence of three throws. Think of it like programming a computer—three throws programmed, three corresponding actions completed, and the activity is finished. However, if you run a pattern, you're repeating the cycle again and again. If I were to ask a juggler to "juggle 441" or "run 441," I'm not asking them to execute those three throws and stop completely. I'm really asking them to do …441441441441441…—running the pattern back-to-back for a period of time.

This might be a little pedantic and heady (okay, it's definitely pretty pedantic and heady), but jugglers use siteswaps both as a kind of programming language (441 = three throws and stop, one cycle of the pattern) as well as a nomenclature—a way to describe the trick as a whole (441 = running the pattern forever, the general idea of 441).

When we refer to 441, it could really mean just one cycle of the pattern (three throws and stopping) or running it ad infinitum. This will be important information later on, especially when we talk about synchronous siteswaps and the way they're written down.

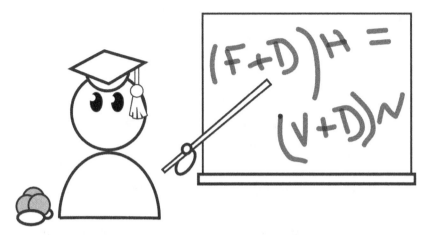

A Mathematical Aside

For my math-inclined friends out there, here's an interesting tool for you. (No, really… you've got to put that Rubik's cube down first, though!) Let's say you see a siteswap that you're unfamiliar with. How do you find out how many objects are in that pattern?[2] To figure this out, you need to find the siteswap's period (that is, the number of throws the pattern has) and the sum of the beats of the pattern (that is, all the beat-values of the throws added together).

Let's use 441 as an example.

441 is period 3—there are three throws in the pattern.
$$4+4+1 = 9$$

Take the sum and divide it by the period to find the number of objects in the pattern: $9/3 = 3$

So, using this formula, we know that 441 is a valid siteswap for three objects.

---

2 This will be explained in greater detail in the next few pages, but know that taking an average does *not* tell you if a pattern is valid!

How about something more complicated?

8448641

Period: 7

Sum: $8+4+4+8+6+4+1 = 35$

Formula: $35/7 = 5$

8448641 is a valid siteswap for five objects. (That means it works!)

Try these out on your own. Are they valid? How many objects are they for?

423

634

75751

88423

97441

8641

But Thom… is this always the case?

You caught me! This is a rule of thumb. Averaging the throws is a necessary but not a sufficient condition to knowing that a pattern is valid. For example, 423 is a valid pattern, but 432 is not. Why is that?

In 423, there are no collisions – each ball lands in a new hand.[3]

In 432, all of the balls end up in the same hand at the same time! It's a mess of collisions.

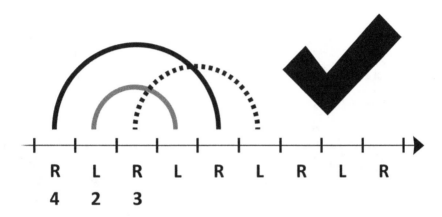

In 423, there are no collisions.

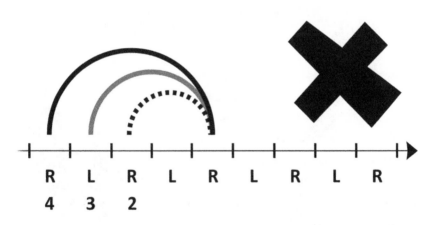

432, however, is a mess of collisions.

If a throw with the value of *n* is immediately followed by *n-1*, for example, you'll have a collision. Same with *n* followed two beats later by *n-2*, and so on.

Synchronous Time

"So, Thom," you say, "that's all well and good. But I like to throw with both hands at the same time!"

An excellent point, friend. The above information pertains to juggling asynchronously—that is, one hand throwing and catching at a time. Siteswap doesn't end there, though! Let's dig in. (C'mon. I saw you pick that Rubik's cube back up!)

When we juggle with a right-hand and left-hand throw at the same time, we're putting two throws into the same beat. In order to note this, we use parentheses and commas. Let's use the four-ball synchronous fountain as an example.

(4,4)

This pattern is called (4,4). When we use synchronous notation, we still mark everything as though it were alternating hands. The hands still alternate as we write them, even though the two throws happen at the same time/on the same beat: (right, left)

Here's another example: (6,4).

In this pattern, nothing crosses. The right hand only juggles 6s and the left hand only

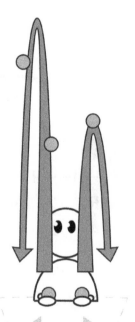

(6,4)

juggles 4s. How do we know how many objects this pattern is for? The parentheses are confusing, but don't let that fool you—the method we used for the asynchronous patterns works here, too:

$$6+4 = 10$$
$$10/2 = 5$$

This is a valid pattern for five balls.

In (6,4), the right hand juggles three balls (thrown at height 6) and the left hand juggles two balls (thrown at height 4.) Simple as that!

But what if we want to get the balls to cross? Let's look at a classic, more complicated five-object pattern:

$$(6x,4)(4,6x)$$

...what does that x mean?

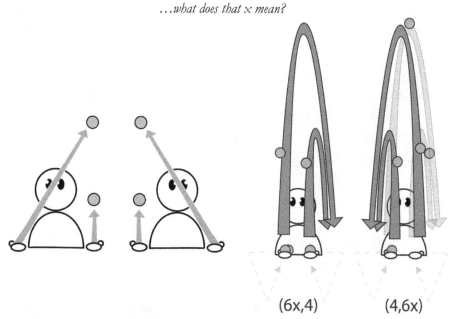

(6x,4)   (4,6x)

(6x,4)*—a five-ball classic. The left illustration is simplified, the right illustration shows accurate flight trajectories.

Since we're lumping two throws into a single beat, we can't have odd-numbered throws in a pattern. There's an excruciatingly nuanced explanation for this. To sum it up, when you have an odd-numbered throw in a synchronous pattern, there's nowhere for the object to land (from the perspective of notation, at least), since we're bundling beats together. In order to mark the idea of a crossing throw, we stick an x behind it. If we didn't, or so I'm told, the space-time continuum would cease to exist. (... and if that happens, it's all your fault!)

(6x,4)(4,6x) is the same series of throws, done from one side to the other—it's a symmetrical pattern, where the throws in each beat are the same, but the hands switch what they're doing. We can simplify the notation, indicating that the throws in the pattern are the same, just switching sides with each beat, by adding an asterisk at the end of the notation when we write it down. That gives us (6x,4)*.

A note about terminology here: If you go to a juggling convention and someone asks you about (6x,4)(4,6x), odds are they'll just say "six ex four" and leave it at that. You'll stand there and scratch your head for a moment—the non-repeating, non-flipped pattern (6x,4) is invalid, after all! When we talk about a pattern that's symmetrical, flipped using an asterisk, jugglers will usually take the easy route and just say the first period of the siteswap.

(...And it should be noted that this is just about the only time you'll find a juggler taking the easy route.)

Multiplexes

Okay, we're getting really, really in deep here. (C'mon. Put that Rubik's cube down. You're gonna need two hands!)

A multiplex is when you throw more than one object from a hand in a single beat. In siteswap, these throws are marked with brackets. (Don't worry about the finer points on actually *making* a multiplex throw—that's all covered in "Multiplex Starts" on page 61). For now, just try to get a feel for what they are and see if you can understand the notation.)

A famous five-ball pattern is called the Gattoplex—named after the famous American juggler Anthony Gatto. This pattern's siteswap is [54]24.

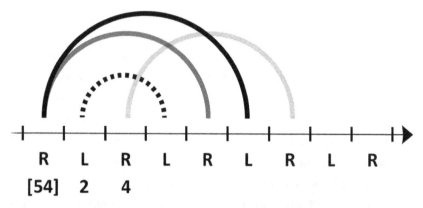

Here, the [54] means that two objects are thrown from one hand at a time. The first to leave the hand is a tall crossing 5, and the other is a 4 which goes slightly lower and returns to the same hand. If you were telling this pattern to another juggler out loud, you'd call it "fifty-four, two, four." (When you say the name of a multiplex out loud, you smash the two throws into one longer number.) This seems really pedantic (and it is), but it's helpful when you're talking siteswap to other jugglers. This is your life now.

Siteswap FAQs

What's the notation for throws that are higher than a 9?

Excellent question! The number after 9 is 10. 10 looks like it could be two throws (1 and 0) or the multiplex [10]. To avoid confusion, we switch to letters after the siteswap 9.

10 is a, 11 is b, 12 is c, and so on.

So, the seven-ball version of the classic three-ball siteswap 531 is db97531. Neat, right?

Does this specific notation work if you only have one hand?

Yes, but…

There are other versions of siteswap that work for different numbers of hands more elegantly than "vanilla" siteswap does. Passers[4] use a four-handed notation[5] as well as something called Prechac Notation.[6] Other multi-handed patterns are possible—as well as a patterns using just one hand.[7] Though you could write an incredible one-handed routine with this notation, you'd need to make some notes to the person you're sharing it with so they'd be able to decode it.

In one-handed siteswap, for example, a 1 is a hold and a 2 is a throw… the notation doesn't change, but the throws look different than a two-handed pattern—no crossing, no hand-switching. The numbers still represent the amount of time an object takes to return to a hand, but that looks a bit different when there's only one hand for the object to return to.

---

4 Passing is juggling with a friend—one big pattern that's spread across everyone's hands. That's a huge topic on its own, and there are a number of resources in print and online about the subject.

5 Four-handed notation is fairly simple if you understand the principles of two-handed notation that we've been going over here. Instead of objects going from Right to Left, the numbers track the objects in a cycle to and from all hands. You can read more about this here: https://www.passingdb.com/articles.php?id=32

6 Prechac looks way more complicated than a "simple" four-handed siteswap—it uses a related, but different method of tracking the length of time objects are in the air. This system is beyond the scope of this little book, but the following article does an excellent job of explaining it: http://www.owenreynolds.net/notation/Symmetric_patterns_C.pdf

7 If you'd like to go down this rabbit hole, check out the following Wikipedia article (as well as its plethora of citations at the end.) https://en.wikipedia.org/wiki/Siteswap#Multi-handed

...That's all outside of the purview of this chapter, however, which only covers vanilla siteswap—which generally comes with the assumption that you're using two hands.

Siteswap Generators

Want more siteswap? No worries at all! Let's let the computers take over here.

There are a number of siteswap generator programs which can help you decipher the patterns appearing in the next appendices. Here are some recommendations which should help you on your way!

Juggling Lab
(Jack Boyce, et al.)

Juggling Lab is a program for Windows and Macintosh that is widely considered to be the best program when it comes to visualizing juggling.

www.jugglinglab.org

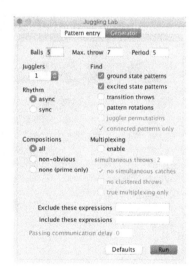

iJuggle (Nathan Peterson)

iJuggle is the best application for Apple phones. It's a beautiful program designed by Nathan Peterson, a programmer who works on juggling robots in his down-time.

www.nathanpeterson.com

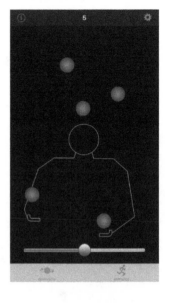

Juggling Lab (Jongle N7)

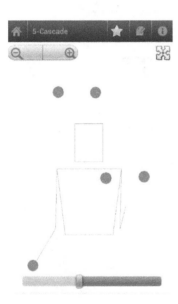

Another classic program, this time for Android devices. This program is based on the original Juggling Lab software, but also allows for passing patterns and other more complicated techniques.

https://play.google.com/store/apps/details?id=com.jonglen7.jugglinglab&hl=en_US

GunSwap (Eric Gunther)

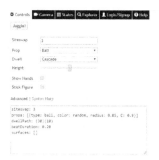

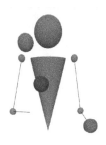

GunSwap is an excellent web-based siteswap generator with a number of parameters that can be altered—including camera angles and more.

www.gunswap.com

APPENDIX B: THE GANDINI SITESWAP LIST

The following is a collection of siteswaps compiled by Matt Hall. The bulk of these come from juggler Sean Gandini's famous DVD *Siteswaps: A Mathematical Juggling Journey*, but many others have contributed to the list.

Special thanks to Sean Gandini and Matt Hall for allowing this compilation's inclusion in this book, with fond memories of Ben Beever.

Three-Ball Siteswaps	5505051	6161601
	61251	6316131
	61305	711
441	61314	7131
423	61350	7401
504	63051	70161
531	63141	70251
5511	63501	70305
51414	64005	70314
51234	64014	70350
52413	64050	70701
52440	64140	72330
52512	64500	73131
53034	66300	73302
53403	6050505	73401
55014	6131451	74130

74400

75300

713151

71701701

801

8040

8130

4| 84012 |2

8123601

6| 9111 |330

45| 90141 |30

5| 9140 |2

45| 90303 |30

45| 90501 |30

Four-Ball Siteswaps

53

552

534

5551

55514

55550

615

633

642

660

6424

61355

62345

62525

62561

63353

63524

63551

63623

64055

64145

64163

64253

64505

64613

64514

66125

61616

66305

66314

66350

6155155

6262525

6461641

71

714

723

741

7126

7333

7405

7441

5| 70166 |3

5| 70256 |3

5| 70355 |3

5| 70364 |3

55| 70616 |2

55| 70625 |2

55| 70661 |1+

56| 70706 |23

5| 72335 |3

5| 72461 |3

73136

73406

73424

72416

72425

73451

73631

74135

5| 74162 |3

74234

74450

74612

74630

5| 75161 |3

75251

75314

75611

7261246

7123456

7161616

7427242

7471414

7272712

7133455

6| 6716071 |33

6| 831 |33

555| 80345 |2

555| 80525 |2

555| 80723 |1

5| 81236 |3

56| 81416 |23

56| 81425 |3

55| 81461 |2

56| 81812 |23

83333

84440

84512

86420

86411

8441841481441

9151

56| 90506 |23

555| 90551 |1

55| 91424 |2

5| 94142 |3

67| 91901 |340

5| 92333 |3

55| 94034 |2

5| 95141 |3

5| 95501 |3

5| 96131 |3

68| a11 |5500

Four-Ball Multiplex and Synch

[43]14

[53]22

[54]21

[43]6421

[53]3423

[54]1424

[54]5123

[54]6122

[64]1324

[64]2323

[64]4123

[65]3123

[74]2421

(4,2x)(4,6x)(6,2)

(2x,4)(6x,4)(2,6)

(8,2)(4x,2x)(2,8)

(2x,4x)

(8,4)(4,2x)(2x,4)

(4,8)(2x,4)(4,2x)

(6x,4)(4,2x)(4,6x)

(2x,4)

Five-Ball Siteswaps

64

645

663

66661

726

744

753

771

7571

7733

7463

74635

72466

73456

74734

75616

75625

75661

75751

6| 75814 |4

77416

77425

77731

6| 777171 |4

747741

66| 825 |3

6| 852 |4

6| 834 |4

66| 861 |3

8633

8246

8273

81277

81475

81727

81772

81817

83446

83833

84445

85246

84733

84742

8448641

8446661

8448551

8537741

8597141

85345

85561

85525

86416

86425

86461

86731

88441

824466

85716814

8558158518551

91

667| 15 |24

7| 933 |44

7| 942 |44

667| 960 |24

90808

92527

67| 92923 |34

94444

94552

94642

667| 95191 |24

95551

95524

67| 96181 |24

96451

96631

67| 96901 |34

97531

94493344

9552952592552

667| a1617 |23

a4448334

a5551a5515a5155a15551

b4a33333

b444b333444

b633633

b447333

d75317531

d5515551

858818151

8558158518551

6| 8851815851 |4

6| 85815815851 |4

66| 9619619169161 |3

678817161

6| 678177171 |4

6| 7718171671 |4

749751714

8648148641

7497517163

94539751714

945397517163

75791571861751

Five-Ball Multiplex and Synch

[53]25

[54]24

[54]1

[43]26

[43]6327

[75]21

[54]6127

[54]7423

[54]6622

[65]1724

[65]2723

[65]6125

[65]3623

[64]4623

[75]3127

[75]3424

[75]5125

[76]3324

[76]4125

[76]3126

[74]4424

[87]33324

[543]24[22]3

[765]3124[22]3

22[43][65]3

22[43][64]4

22[54][65]1

22[64][64]1

[987]313124[22]3

555524[74]445555

555524[84]444555

555524[94]444455

555524[22]3[764]7161555

555524[22]3[764]81716714

555524[22]3[654]6155555

555524[22]3[654]7145555

555524[22]3[765]3155555

555524[22]3[987]3131555

(6x,4)(6,4x)

(6x,4)(4,6x)

(6,4)(6x,4)(4,6)(4,6x)

(6,4x)(6,4)(4x,6)(4,6)

(6x,4x)(6,4x)(4x,6x)(4x,6)

(8,2x)(2x,8)

(8x,2x)(6,4x)(2x,8x)(4x,6)

(8x,4)(4x,6x)(6x,2x)*

Six-Ball Siteswaps

774

756

855

864

7| 945 |5

7| 963 |5

9645

9555

85845

94944

99192

96456

96627

96852

b55555

b97531

8686716

9595881771

Six-Ball Multiplex and Synch

[54]27

[65]25

[75]24

[76]23

[65]7246

[54]6627

[65]6625

[75]5625

[76]4625

[76]7226

[76]4724

[87]4425

[54][75]522

27[543]

(8x,6)(4,6x)*

Seven-Ball Siteswaps

966

948

b6666

8888881

9797971

[75]27

[86]25

[54][65]1

[43][65]3

[43][64]4

[64][64]1

[86][86]322

[987]4426[22]5

[7654]26[22]5[222]4

APPENDIX C: TYPES OF JUGGLING BALLS

There are three main types of juggling balls: the beanbag, the russian, and the stage ball.

Beanbags

Beanbags are the simplest and most popular style of juggling ball. They're usually made from a fabric shell and filled with millet. These can range from a few dollars per ball to $20 per ball—it all depends on the number of panels, kind of filling, and type of fabric that's used.

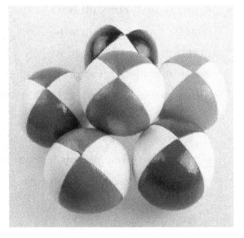

Many professional jugglers use beanbags made from leather or ultrasuede, since they last a long time. Beginner and intermediate jugglers often use beanbags made with vinyl, since they don't take long to break in, can take a lot of abuse, and are relatively inexpensive.

The advantage of beanbags is that they don't roll very far when you drop them. They're also available in a wide range of colors, weights, and sizes.

Russians

The Russian juggling ball is a plastic shell that's partly filled with sand or salt. These were invented in the 1970s by a Ukranian juggler named Mikhail Rudenko (Vysotskyi, 2016).

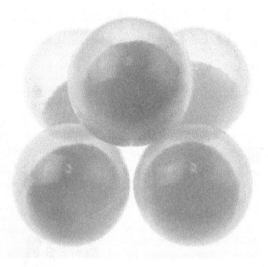

Russians feel strange to juggle at first, but with time many people prefer them to beanbags. The advantage to Russians is their "dead drop"—when they hit the ground, they stay put. This also makes some body stalls easier (catching on the elbow, the foot, etc.)

Russians are easy and cheap to make on your own or relatively inexpensive to buy pre-made from many online shops. If you'd like to learn to make these, check out the next chapter!

Stage Balls

Stage balls are a hollow plastic shell, made from thick plastic or vinyl. These are great for rolling on the body as a contact juggling ball, and they look great in the air. They are unforgiving when you drop, though, and have a tendency to roll.

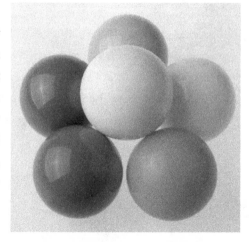

Bounce Balls

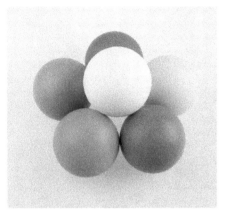

Bounce juggling balls are made of a variety of different materials, the most common being rubber.

In older days, the "gold standard" bounce ball was the silicon ball—an expensive prop, but with an incredible natural rebound. Today, however, a number of companies have discovered new ways to increase the rebound of simple rubber balls which has led to many very good, very inexpensive props for aspiring bounce jugglers.

If you're curious about learning to juggle by throwing balls at the ground, pick up a set and see what you can do! These are, of course, perfectly compatible with toss juggling in the air—just watch out for collisions!

Of course, there are a number of other hybrid styles of juggling balls—shells filled with liquid, stage balls with millet, rubber balls that bounce, and more. Everyone has their own preferences… and with time, you'll probably have a favorite style of ball, too!

Check out your local juggling club and try out a variety of styles.

Ball images courtesy of Tom Kidwell, Renegade Juggling.

APPENDIX D: DIY JUGGLING BALLS

Haec quae de facili turget paganica pluma,

folle minus est et minus arta pila.

This paganica ball that swells with yeilding feathers,

is not so soft as the inflated balls, nor so hard as the handballs.

- Martial, *Epigrams*, 10.45

FIRST AND FOREMOST, the best prop is the one you've got. The only way to get better at juggling is with practice! The poor carpenter blames his tools, and if there were a style or brand of juggling ball that would make you the best juggler in the world, this book wouldn't be necessary. That said, there are some qualities in balls that are more favorable than others—the ideal juggling ball, if your author's opinion carries any weight to, is about 70 millimeters in diameter and weighs around 120 grams.

If you don't have the cash to buy a ball made specifically for juggling, let's look at some ways to make a prop that's better than the balled-up socks you've been practicing with.

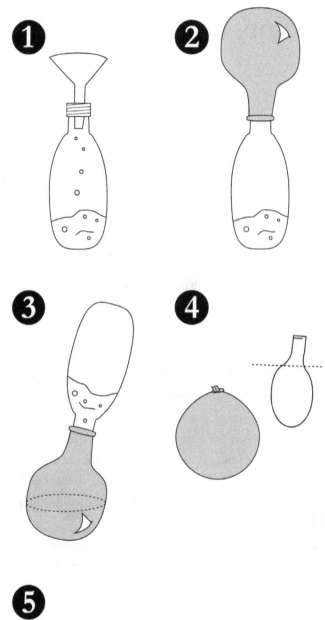

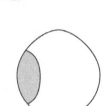

Balloons and Birdseed

THESE BALLS ARE A summer-camp classic. When I used to teach juggling at the YMCA in Colorado, these were the props we used. They're simple, reliable, and relatively sturdy. It can be difficult to make a set of balls that all have the same exact weight with this method, but you can still get close and make something that's great to learn with.

What you need:
- A clean (and dry!) 2-liter bottle
- Balloons (helium-quality are ideal)
- Birdseed (avoid seed mixes that contain sunflower seeds. They're sharp and can rupture the balloons)
- A sharp pair of scissors
- A funnel

1. Use the funnel to fill the bottle with your seed mix.

2. Inflate the balloon about twice the size of your desired juggling ball size. Then stretch its nozzle over the top of the bottle. You will lose some air from the balloon while doing this, and that's okay.

3. Turn the bottle over and fill the balloon with your desired amount of seed.

4. Tie off the balloon that's now filled with seeds. Take another balloon and cut it just below its "shoulder," where the nozzle goes from straight to round.

5. Wrap the cut balloon around the one filled with seed. Try to make sure the seed-filled balloon's nozzle is covered with the exterior cut balloon.

6. You're done! Now make a few more and go practice!

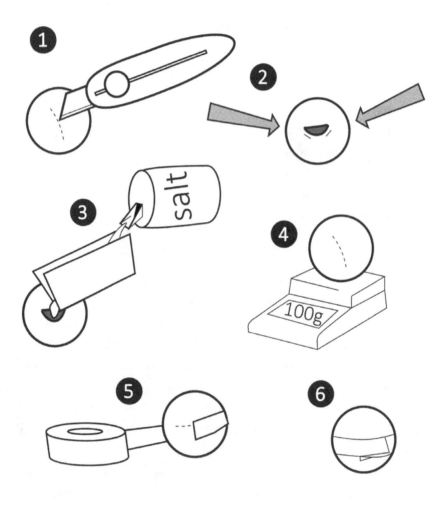

Russians

These balls are an excellent prop to work with. In fact, many professional jugglers use home-made, russian-style balls instead of buying something from a retailer!

What you need:
• Hollow-shell play pit balls (easily found in the baby or toy section at Target, Walmart, etc.)
• A sharp knife (X-Acto, razor blade, etc.)
• A container of salt or sand (make sure it's dry!)
• A scale
• Electrical tape
• An index card

1. Cut a small incision in the side of the play pit balls. I usually make a cut that's about 1/2 - 3/4 inch in length. Too short, and you'll have a hard time filling it. Too long, and you'll have a hard time sealing it.

2. Squeeze the sides of the balls to make the incisions pucker.

3. Fold your index card, place its corner next to an incision, and pour salt into the ball.

4. Weigh the ball and see how close you are to your target weight. Add more salt or take some out if needed.

5. Tightly wrap electrical tape over the incision, wrapping the tape all around the ball's latitude.

6. Cut the tape and make sure it's sealed. Then make some more and go practice!

Other Balls That Work Well for Juggling

Don't want to take on another project? That's all right! There are a ton of everyday balls that are good for learning.

The standard juggling ball on the market today ranges from 62-72 millimeters—that's about 2.5 inches to 3.25 inches in diameter—with a weight between 80 and 150 grams. If you don't have a way to buy balls made specifically for juggling, there are a few types of balls that you can find in just about any sports shop that will work.

Lacrosse balls

These work in a pinch but aren't ideal for the absolute beginner, as they bounce when they're dropped. If you go with these, think about juggling over thick carpet, a bed, or grass so you won't have to chase after them.

Baseballs

Baseballs have a great weight to them, though they might be too big for learners with smaller hands. (Softballs are way too big!) These are extremely durable, but thanks to their hard leather shell, they can also be punishing to your hands and fingertips.

Tennis Balls (modified)

Tennis balls straight from the court are too light for juggling, but have a good size. These can be turned into russians, filled up entirely with pennies, or injected with water to make a suitable juggling ball.

APPENDIX E: JUGGLING WARM-UPS

Drill for Accuracy—The Growing Pattern

This is a very popular warm-up for technical jugglers. In fact, the in-joke at the International Jugglers' Association festival is about this drill. If you see a juggler standing still and juggling three balls very high... odds are, they're extremely good.[27]

Here's how it works: Stand in one spot and juggle three balls, gradually throwing higher and higher. This sounds simple at first, but it can be a very sobering drill that forces you to focus on total precision and accuracy with your throw heights.

Start by planting your feet (shoulder width!) and juggling three balls in a cascade. Once you achieve 10 to 20 catches, it's time to start increasing the height. Bring the pattern up taller—slowly—to the height of a five-ball cascade. For now, think about keeping the rhythm of the pattern even and measured. Once you achieve 10 to 20 catches, it's time to bring the pattern up to a seven-ball cascade height. Continue with this progression until you reach the ceiling (or drop!).

When you feel comfortable with this exercise, take the pattern up toward the ceiling and then bring it back down with the same control and accuracy.

This drill is important for a few reasons. If you can't juggle three balls at a seven-ball height, how well will you juggle seven balls at a seven-ball height? (Not well at all!) This drill allows you to "check in" with your hands, arms, and shoulders before you start a real training session. It helps you identify issues with your accuracy in a kind of technical

---

27 ...and if you see a juggler doing this drill with a single ball, odds are they're Ukrainian!

vacuum—the skill you're performing here isn't technically difficult, so it allows you to see if one hand is throwing too far forward, outside, behind you, etc. This allows you to adjust your technique before you begin working on new patterns and techniques.

Be mindful of how you move to make stray catches: if you walk, if you tend to put more weight in one foot than the other, etc. This drill allows you to shine a spotlight on your technique and identify and correct any issues you discover.

If this drill is getting too simple for you (or if you just want to mix things up!), feel free to adjust the rhythm. Instead of a slow and measured three balls, try working on it in flashes where all three balls are being thrown quickly—siteswap 7770000 instead of 720720720.

Hand and Shoulder Warm-ups—T. Rex & Hand Slaps

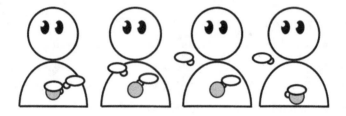

The claw-catching game is one of my absolute favorites. I use this as a warm-up for most of my session classes at circus schools. I also lifted this warmup shamelessly from Yuri Pozdnyakov, the head juggling instructor at the circus school in Kiev, Ukraine.

Take a single ball and hold it in your hand. Imagine you are a Tyrannosaurs rex. Or a pianist, or a T. rex that learned to play the piano. Hold your hands like that—with the elbows tucked in touching your sides and your forearms perpendicular to the vertical axis of your spine. Your hands are near the line of your navel. Your palms are facing down. Now, move your forearms so your hands are touching in front of you, at your center line, approximately the height of your navel. (Make sure that your elbows are still touching your sides—the movement that positions your hands along the center line comes from the humerus and shoulder.)

Now, lift your hand up and release the ball so it drifts upward toward the height of the lowest part of your sternum, moving that hand up and out of the way upon release. With the opposite hand, claw-catch the ball and assume the original posture. Repeat this, going faster and faster. With some practice, it will eventually look like the ball is simply floating in the air along the axis of your center line. Be sure to maintain the original posture with your elbows touching your sides—you'll start to feel your shoulders and forearms working.

Check in with your hands as well—the ball should not spin as it is released. The release should be sharp and quick, with your hand simply opening up and letting the ball drop as it is lifted up.

Once you have achieved some success with this drill (or simply gotten bored with it!), re-square your arms and elbows, this time with the palms of your hands facing each other, about shoulder-width apart. (Imagine holding a large box in front of you, with your hands on opposite sides of the box.)

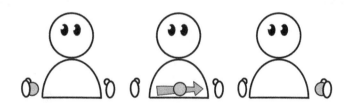

Throw the ball from one hand to the other, going faster and faster. This throw is directly across, like a laser. When you make the throw, be sure your hands never cross the center line of your body.

When you feel ready, pass the ball right to left in front of your body, and left to right behind your back—the ball circles your waist like a hula-hoop or a moon in rapid orbit around you.

What next? Alternate directions! Go in circles! Be sure you keep your elbows static and only move the entire apparatus of your arm with the shoulder muscles.

The important thing here is that we're isolating the muscles of our shoulders' rotator cuffs and waking them up.

Feel the burn? Congrats! You're done with this warm-up!

Legendary jugglers Paul Ponce and Gena Shvartsman Cristiani offer a different hand warmup. This one is strange, but they both declared its efficacy in a panel discussion at the 2017 International Jugglers' Association festival in Cedar Rapids, Iowa.

Put your hands back in the pianist/T. rex position once again, centered toward the navel, only this time with loose wrists. Move one hand above the other and—*slap!* Bring the top hand down and slap the lower hand, moving down and through the lower hand. Now, your hands are in the reverse position from the first. Bring the top hand down and strike the other one.

Repeat this until your hands feel warm and ready to go, it hurts too much to continue, or you start getting strange looks from the people around you.

A Comprehensive List of Total Body Warm-ups for Jugglers

Some people skip rope.

APPENDIX F: GLOSSARY

Asynchronous Time	The hands move on alternating beats.
Beat	An arbitrary measurement of time used in siteswap notation.
Center Line	A line going from navel to nose and further on up into space and time. Objects cross from one hand to the other at a point on the center line. Balances also happen along the center line.
Center of Gravity	The point of equilibrium of an object that is being balanced. On a broomstick, this would be the exact midpoint of the length of the stick. On a hammer, juggling club, or broom handle with the bristles still attached, this point would be much closer to the heavy end of the object.
Corner	A place above the shoulder where an object begins its descent.
Flash	A single cycle of juggling throws, equal to the number of objects being manipulated. A three-ball flash is three throws and three catches of a three-ball cascade.
Internal Metronome	A juggler's natural cadence.
Inside Throw	A "vanilla" throw—the basic throw in a juggling pattern. These throws travel along the path of a standard scooping motion, from the outside to the release point on the inside of the shoulder.

Multiplex	A throw where multiple objects are released from the same hand at the same time.
Pattern	A series of throws done in succession that repeats. The basic three-ball cascade is a pattern. So is a sequence of throws under the leg, if it repeats.
Picture Plane	The two-dimensional representation of what you see with your eyes. The "picture plane of vision" is like a painting of what you see without considering depth of field.
Qualify	Two cycles of juggling throws, double the number of objects being manipulated. A three-ball qualify is six throws and six catches of a three-ball cascade.
Rainbow Throw	A reverse throw, where the object travels in a scoop moving outward. These throws peak on the same side as the hand that released them, rather than the corner opposite the throwing hand.
Sequence	A series of throws or catches that do not necessarily repeat indefinitely; a piece of choreography.
Siteswap	A mathematical system for recording juggling patterns. The numbers in siteswap represent the duration of time, measured in beats, that it takes for an object to return to a hand.
Synchronous Time	When the hands move on the same beats.
Vanilla	Basic; standard; the most stripped-down version. Nothing fancy; no embellishments.
Vanilla Siteswap	Uncomplicated patterns in asynchronous time (right, left, right, left...).

APPENDIX G: RECOMMENDED READING: THE NEXT STEP

Finished this book and ready for more? Here's a selection of titles and thoughts about when you should tuck into them.

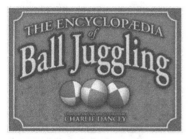

Three-Ball Tricks

Charlie Dancey's Encyclopaedia of Ball Juggling
Charlie Dancey, Butterfingers Press
ISBN 978-1898591139

Four-Ball Tricks

Four Ball Juggling—From simple patterns to advanced theory
Martin Probert, Self-published
ISBN 978-0952486008

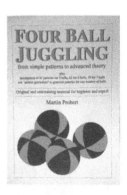

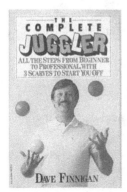

Other Juggling Props

The Complete Juggler
Dave Finnigan, Vintage Books
ISBN 978-0394746784

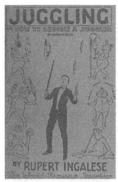

Juggling: or how to become a juggler (annotated edition)
Rupert Ingalese, Modern Vaudeville Press
ISBN 978-1733971201

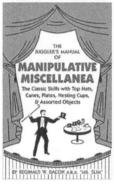

The Juggler's Book of Manipulative Miscellanea
Reginald Bacon, Variety Arts Press
ISBN 978-0981794518

More on Siteswap

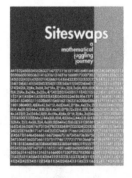

Siteswaps (DVD)
Sean Gandini, et al., Media Circus
Social Juggling

Juggling History

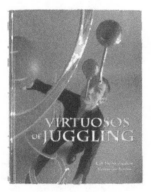

Virtuosos of Juggling
Karl-Heinz Ziethen, Renegade Juggling
ISBN 978-0974184807

Headier Topics

Tactile
Luke Wilson, Gandini Press
ISBN 978-0-9955024-2-0

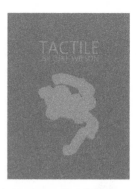

5 Catches
Jay Gilligan, Blurb.com
No ISBN

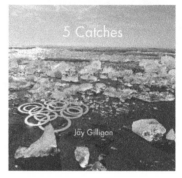

Other Resources

www.juggle.org
www.jugglingedge.com
www.historicaljugglingprops.com
www.renegadejuggling.com
www.playjuggling.com
www.henrys-online.de
www.circustalk.com
www.circopedia.org
www.libraryofjuggling.com

BIBLIOGRAPHY

Åberg, E. (2018, April 15). (T. Wall, Interviewer).

Amazeen, E. L., Amazeen, P. G., Post, A. A., & Beek, P. J. (1999). Timing the selection of information during rhythmic catching. *Journal of Motor Behavior* (31), 279-289.

Bacrach, Fontbonne, Joufflineau, and Ulloa. (2015). "Audience entrainment during live contemporary dance performance: physiological and cognitive measures". *Frontiers in Human Neuroscience* (9). 179.

Byrne, P., & Crawford, J. (2010). Cue reliability and a landmark stability heuristic determine relative weighting between egocentric and allocentric visual information in memory-guided reach. *Journal of Neurophysiology*, 3054-3069.

Catanzariti, J. (1998). A Comparison of Two Methods for Teaching Three-Ball Juggling. https://minds.wisconsin.edu/bitstream/handle/1793/22057/Catanzariti.pdf?sequence=1&isAllowed=y

Cavanagh, P., & Alvarez, G. (2005). Tracking multiple targets with multifocal attention. *Trends in Cognitive Science*, 349-354.

Chandler, A. (1991). On the Symbolism of Juggling: The Moral and Aesthetic Implications of the Mastery of Falling Objects. *Journal of Popular Culture*, 25(3). Retrieved from http://www.juggling.org/papers/symbolism/#fn1

Cinquevalli, P. (1909, 3). How to Succeed as a Juggler. *Cassell's Magazine*, 47(4).

Dessing, J. C., Frederic, R. P., & Beek, P. J. (2011, December 6). Gaze fixation improves the stability of expert juggling. *Experimental*

Brain Research. Retrieved from https://www.ncbi.nlm.nih.gov/pmc/articles/PMC3268979/

Draganski, B., Gaser, C., Busch, V., Schuierer, G., & Bogdahn, U. (2004). Changes in grey matter induced by training. Neuroplasticity: *Nature*, 311-312.

Haibach, P., Daniels, G., & Newell, K. (2004). Coordination changes in the early stages of learning to cascade juggle. *Human Movement Science*, 185-206.

Leigh, R., & Zee, D. (2006). *The neurology of eye movements*. New York: Oxford Press.

Meltzer, S. (2012, July 14). Thou Shalt Not Steal. Retrieved from *eJuggle*: http://www.juggle.org/be-funnier-with-scotty-meltzer-thou-shalt-not-steal/

Morisita, M., & Yagi, T. (2001). The stability of human eye orientation during visual fixation and imagined fixation in three dimensions. *Auris Nasus Larynx*, 301-304.

Morita, Y., Ogawa, K., & Uchida, S. (2016). Napping after complex motor learning enhances juggling performance. *Sleep Science*, 112-116. Retrieved from https://www.ncbi.nlm.nih.gov/pmc/articles/PMC5021952/

Rodrigues, S., Polastri, P. F., Gotardi, G., & Barbieri, F. (2016, 8). Postural Control During Cascade Ball Juggling: Effects of Expertise and Base of Support. *Perceptual and Motor Skills*, 279-294.

Sanchez Garcia, R., Hayes, S. J., Williams, A. M., & Bennett, S. J. (2013). Multisensory Perception and Action in 3-Ball Cascade Juggling. *Journal of Motor Behavior*, 29-36. Retrieved from https://slides.tips/multisensory-perception-and-action-in-3-ball-cascade-juggling.html#

Táin Bó Cúailnge. (2002). (T. Kinsella, Trans.) Oxford University Press.

Vysotskyi, S. (2016, 10 30). Mikhail Rudenko, inventor of Russian Balls. Retrieved from *eJuggle*: https://www.juggle.org/mikhail-rudenko-inventor-of-russian-balls/

SPECIAL THANKS

215 Festival*

Will Andreas

Dan Barron

Becky Brown

Blue Stoop*

David Cain

Benjamin Domask-Ruh

Luke Emery

Jackie Erikson

Judy Finelli

Kathleen Finneran

Sean Gandini

Megan Gendell

Jay Gilligan

Fritz Grobe

Matt Hall

Jim Hendricks

Madeline Hoak

Maika Isogawa

Richard Kennison

Tom Kidwell

Gregor Kiok

Marysia Kochać

Kate Peterson Koch

Sophie Lewis

Sam Malcolm

Scotty Meltzer

Jon Monastero

Mike Moore

Philadelphia Performance Artists' Emergency Fund

Avi Pryntz-Nadworny

Andrew Olson

Denis Paumier

Kate Peterson Koch

The Philadelphia Writers Emergency Fund*

Matan Presberg

Eric Shibuya

Chase Davidson Smith

Sam Veale

Nathan Wakefield

Jon Wee

*Indicates a financial contribution from the Philadelphia Writers Emergency Fund, offering relief for writers affected by the COVID-19 crisis.

ABOUT THE AUTHORS

Benjamin Domask-Ruh

Benjamin Domask-Ruh is a circus and theatre director, performer, and clown who resides in Minnesota and works all around the world.

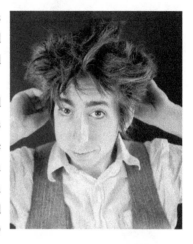

His work has been experienced throughout the United States as a performer and teacher with the International Jugglers' Association (2014 - present), touring actor with Tigerlion Arts (2017), commissioned playwright for CLIMB Theatre (2019 - present,) principle juggler with MOTH Poetic Circus (2018 - 2019,) Assistant Director with Children's Theatre Company in Minneapolis, Minnesota (2019), and a guest instructor with youth circuses such as Circus Harmony, Trenton Circus Squad, and Circus Juventas (2012 - Present).

Internationally, Benjamin tours with longtime Modern Vaudeville partner Thom Wall with their award-winning juggling show, "The 'Dinner and a Show' Show;" as well as with circus partner Timmyto Bond in Mexico. Benjamin also performs his solo show, "HODGE PODGE," across North America. Benjamin is a proud Teaching Artist of St. Paul based COMPAS and is professionally managed by Afton Benson.

Benjamin is also the pedagogic editor of the book you're holding in your hands and the model for the LED juggling illustrations.

Jay Gilligan

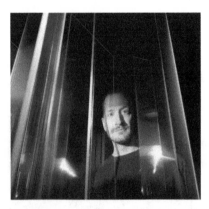

Jay Gilligan has performed in 33 different countries, touring solo work and collaborating with companies such as The Gandini Juggling Project, Cie Jérôme Thomas, Les 7 doigts de la main, Cirkus Cirkör, and Cirque du Soleil. He has been a juggling teacher at every major circus school in the world and published a book about contemporary juggling titled *5 Catches*. Most recently, Jay collaborated with Cie Ea Eo to create a juggling ceremony which will welcome aliens to Earth, should they ever visit this planet.

Fritz Grobe

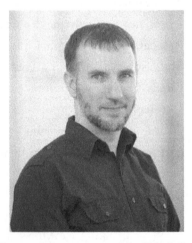

Fritz Grobe has over 30 years' experience as a professional performer, creative director, and choreographer for award-winning circus acts and stage performances. As a juggler, he has won five gold medals at the International Jugglers' Association Festival and set a world record for bounce juggling way too many objects.

He was artistic director of the juggling and dance ensemble "blink," which toured North America and Europe for five years (with Jay Gilligan from 1995-1996 and with Morten Hansen from 1995-2000) and won the International Jugglers' Association Team Championships in Las Vegas.

He was a lead actor and the featured solo clown in the original cast of Cirque Mechanics' "Birdhouse Factory," and he is the co-founder of Eepybird Studios, best known for their viral videos featuring the explosive combination of Diet Coke and Mentos, that have been viewed over 150 million times. Their work has won four Webby Awards and two Emmy nominations.

He has appeared on *The Late Show with David Letterman*, *Mythbusters*, *Ellen*, *The Today Show*, and more, and performed live in London, Paris, Istanbul, New York, Las Vegas, Oslo, Cairo, Xi'an, and Tokyo.

For more than 20 years and 200+ performances, Fritz has also been a writer and performer for "The Early Evening Show," Maine's longest-running live variety show, at Celebration Barn Theater in South Paris, Maine.

Thom Wall

Thom Wall is an American juggler who specializes in learning juggling tricks from the past. He has performed in 17 countries on four continents, including a run of his solo history show, "On the Topic of Juggling,"

at the Smithsonian Institution in Washington, D.C. The digital version of his book *Juggling: From Antiquity to the Middle Ages* was awarded "Best Nonfiction Title" by the Indie Book Awards in 2019.

Thom also performed as a solo act with Cirque du Soleil's touring big-top show *Totem* from 2014 - 2019.

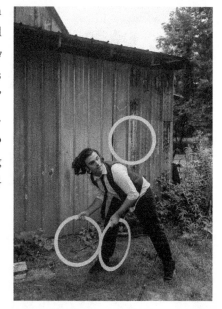

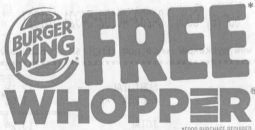

Burger King ®
BK 13948

3 Cedar Swamp Road
Glen Cove, New York
516-609-0813

ORDER 20

DRIVE THRU

1	CHK NUGGETS 10PC	1.00
1	CMLG BACON KING	11.19
1	*BACON KING	
	1 PLAIN	
1	*LG FRY	
1	*LG COKE ZERO	

****

Free WHOPPER Sandwich or
Original Chicken Sandwich
Purchase required

Survey Code: 04232-40102-54921-181827

www.mybkexperience.com (English or Espanol)
****

SUBTOTAL	12.19
8.625% TAX	1.05
TOTAL	13.24
CASH	20.00
CHANGE	6.76

QUESTIONS COMMENTS?
PLEASE VISIT WWW.MYBKEXPERIENCE.COM
Mon Dec 24 2018 08:54 PM T=10L I=5 C=103

Other Books by Modern Vaudeville Press

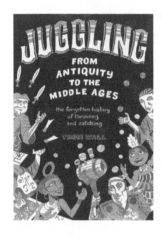

Juggling: From Antiquity to the Middle Ages
Thom Wall
ISBN 978-0-578-41084-5

As with dance, so with juggling—the moment that the performer finishes the routine, their act ceases to exist beyond the memory of the audience. There is no permanent record of what transpired, so studying the ancient roots of juggling is fraught with difficulty. Using the records that do exist, juggling appears to have emerged around the world in cultures independent of one another in the ancient past. Paintings in Egypt from 2000 BCE show jugglers engaged in performance. Stories from the island nation of Tonga place juggling's creation with their goddess of the underworld—a figure who has guarded a cave since time immemorial. Juggling games and rituals are pervasive in isolated Inuit cultures in northern Canada and Greenland. Though the earliest representation of juggling is 4,000 years old, the practice is surely much older—in the same way that humans were doubtlessly singing and dancing long before the first bone flute was created.

This book is an attempt to catalogue this tangible history of juggling in human culture. It is the story of juggling, represented in art and writing from around the world, across time. Although much has been written about modern jugglers–specific performers, their props, and their routines–little has been said about those who first developed the craft. As juggling enters a golden age in the internet era, Juggling: From Antiquity to the Middle Ages offers a look into the past—to the origins of our art form.

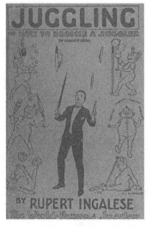

Juggling: or How to Become a Juggler (the annotated edition)
Rupert Ingalese, Thom Wall
ISBN 978-1733971201

Rupert Ingalese, born Paul Wingrave, was a British juggler who worked in the first half of the 1900s, both as a juggler and as a producer and manager of variety shows across England. In 1917, he published the very first "learn to juggle" book, teaching in detail the methods used to learn traditional toss juggling as well as a variety of more esoteric juggling skills.

This edition offers complete annotations that add context to Ingalese's writing as well as asides that explain the work of other jugglers in the same time period.

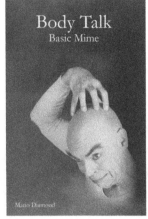

Body Talk: Basic Mime
Mario Diamond
ISBN 978-1-7339712-1-8

Body Talk is Mario Diamond's detailed introduction to the art of mime. Body axes, illusions, and exploratory games are laid out accessibly for any learner.

The Midwest Book Review calls this book "...a highly recommended 'must' for any theater or drama reference collection and for producers and actors who want to translate mime's basics to better acting and cognitive results."

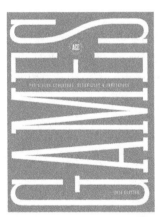

Games for Circus Educators, Organizers &
Innovators
American Youth Circus Organization, compiled by Lucy Little
ISBN 978-1-7339712-2-5

With over 100 games organized for optimal use in cooperative, movement-based settings, this book is a must-have for every circus school, teaching artist, and arts education program! Games are organized by age, number of participants, energy level, and social/emotional learning outcome, and include special notes for working with a variety of populations that may require adaptation or modifications.

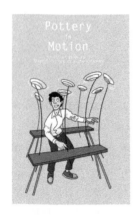

Pottery in Motion: A practical guide to the impractical art of plate spinning
Sam Veale
ISBN 978-1-7339712-3-2

Judging by the books already available with the words "Plate Spinning" in the title, there is a good chance that you picked this up because you are a working parent trying to balance your home life with a busy career. If so, I can't help you. This book deals with plate spinning in the strictly literal sense. Unless you are interested in spinning ceramic plates on sticks, I won't waste any more of your precious time, save to say, best of luck with the kids and the job.

If you are actually interested in spinning actual plates on actual sticks, then this is the book for you (but if you end up struggling to balance your home life with your busy career as a plate spinner, then don't say I didn't warn you).

FREE E-BOOK!

If you enjoyed *Juggling: What It Is and How to Do It*, you might be interested in *What Scientists Have to Say About Juggling*: A 15-page treatise on the current state of juggling research. This Amazon bestselling booklet outlines juggling and its effects on the practitioner's body and mind.

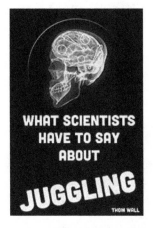

Now available as a free digital download!
http://thomwall.com/sciencebook

"The nerdiest non-nerdy explanation of the current state of juggling research in the world. Super legit content, mixed with light touch of humor."

Craig Quat: www.quatprops.com

"This ebook covers an incredible amount of research while keeping the information engaging and useful for a juggling practice. I have been either training, performing, or teaching juggling for about two decades, and I learned a ton! Whether you're just discovering an interest in juggling or you're far down the rabbit hole, read this today."

Jeremy Fein: www.feinmovement.com

"This paper is in-depth, interesting, and informative. Thom has dug up some of the juiciest academic and scientific tidbits of our art to help legitimize and de-stigmatize the word "juggler." Time spent reading this book will not only deeply intrigue the casual reader but help facilitate the education potentials of teachers and hobbyists alike."

Benjamin Domask: www.benjamindomask.com

CPSIA information can be obtained
at www.ICGtesting.com
Printed in the USA
BVHW030028130920
588727BV00001B/300